AF266847

ARTHRITIS

A Doctor's Practical Guide to Pain Control & Mobility

Dr Prabhat Das
MD, PhD, FACP

Better Health with Dr Das Series

Hardcover ISBN: 978-1-971672-58-8

Paperback ISBN: 978-1-971672-57-1

eBook ISBN: 978-1-971672-56-4

Printed in the United States of America

Disclaimer

This book is intended solely for educational and informational purposes. It is not meant to replace personal medical advice, diagnosis, or treatment.

Although I am a licensed physician, reading this book does not establish a doctor-patient relationship. Each individual's health condition, medical history, and risk factors are unique. Any medical decision should be made in partnership with your own healthcare professional who understands your specific situation.

Medical science is continually advancing. New research and updated guidelines may lead to changes in recommendations over time.

TABLE OF CONTENTS:

About the Author

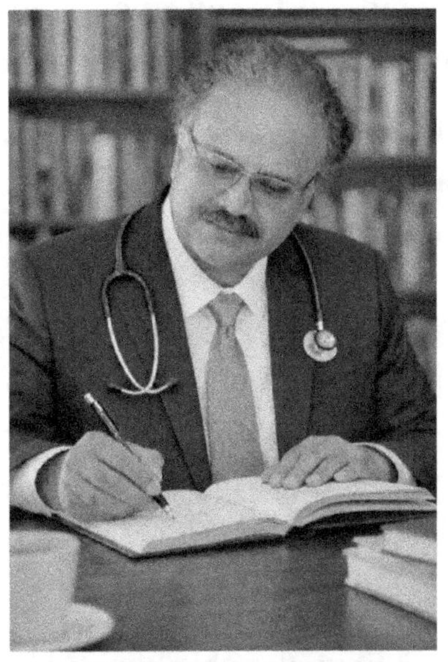

I am Dr Prabhat Das, MD, PhD, FACP. My journey in medicine began in India and, over the past thirty-five years, has continued in the United States, where I have had the privilege of caring for patients across a wide range of medical settings. I am trained in Internal Medicine, Pulmonary Diseases, and Critical Care. For me, medicine has never been just a profession. It has been a lifelong commitment shaped by learning, service, and a deep respect for the trust patients place in their physician.

Over the years, I have had the honor of caring for patients in many different situations. I have seen individuals in my office for routine concerns, treated urgent conditions in busy emergency rooms, managed serious illnesses in the hospital, and cared for critically ill patients in intensive care units. Each setting has taught me something valuable. Each patient has added to my understanding of what it truly means to care for another human being.

But one lesson has stood above all others. Medicine is not only about tests, diagnoses, or treatments. It is about people. It is about listening carefully, understanding fears that are often left unspoken, and guiding patients through uncertainty with clarity and compassion. Again and again, I have seen that what people want most is simple, trustworthy information. They want to understand what is happening in their bodies. They want to feel confident about the decisions they are making for their health and for their families.

These experiences have deeply shaped how I think about health, illness, prevention, and the human side of healing.

That is the reason behind the '**<u>Better Health with Dr Das Series</u>'.** Through these books, I hope to reach individuals I may never meet in person but who are searching for clear and reliable guidance. In today's world, health information is everywhere, yet much of it is confusing, overwhelming, and sometimes misleading. My goal is to cut through that noise and present important medical topics in a way that is simple, practical, and reassuring.

Every page of this series is guided by two foundations: reliable scientific knowledge and decades of real-world clinical experience. I want you, the reader, to feel informed, confident, and empowered. Not overwhelmed. Not confused. But clear about what you can do, step by step, to improve your health.

If even one reader feels less anxious, more informed, or better prepared to take control of their health after reading these books, then this work has served its purpose.

Helping people live healthier, longer, more confident and better-informed lives remains one of the greatest privileges of my life.

CHAPTER 1: Arthritis Explained Simply

Why This Book Matters

In my daily practice, I hear this sentence again and again:

"Doctor, I think I have arthritis."

It sounds simple. But it is not.

Behind that one word lies a wide range of conditions, experiences, and outcomes. For one person, it may mean a dull ache in the knee while climbing stairs. For another, it may be stiff fingers every morning. For someone else, it may be sudden, severe pain in a single joint that makes even the lightest touch unbearable.

That is why arthritis must be understood clearly and carefully.

This book is written with a simple goal. I want to remove confusion. I want to give you clarity. When you understand your condition, you begin to feel more in control. And when you feel more in control, your decisions improve, and so do your results.

Arthritis Is Not One Disease

One of the most important things to understand from the
beginning is this:

Arthritis is not a single disease.

It is a broad term used to describe a group of conditions
that affect the joints and surrounding tissues. There are
many types, each with different causes, patterns, and
treatments.

Most people use the word "arthritis" as if it means only
wear and tear of joints. That is only one part of the story.

Some types are related to gradual joint wear. Others are
caused by inflammation. Some are due to crystal
deposits. A few may be related to infection or systemic
illness.

This difference matters.

Because treatment depends on the cause.

What Exactly Is a Joint?

Before we go further, let us understand what a joint is.

A joint is where two bones meet. These joints allow you to
move, bend, walk, lift, and perform daily activities.

Think about how many joints you use in a single day:

- Knees when you walk
- Hips when you sit and stand

- Fingers when you write or hold objects
- Shoulders when you reach or lift

When joints are healthy, you do not even notice them. They work quietly in the background.

When they become painful or stiff, they begin to affect everything.

What Happens in Arthritis?

The word arthritis literally means **inflammation of a joint**.

But in practice, arthritis can involve more than inflammation.

Depending on the type, there may be:

- Wear and thinning of cartilage
- Swelling of the joint lining
- Accumulation of fluid
- Formation of crystals
- Damage to surrounding structures

The result is often similar:

- Pain
- Stiffness
- Swelling
- Reduced movement

But the underlying cause may be very different.

And that is why identifying the type is essential.

Arthritis Is Not Just "Aging"

Many people believe arthritis is simply a part of growing older.

There is some truth to this, but it is not the complete picture.

Certain types, especially osteoarthritis, become more common with age. But arthritis is not an inevitable or harmless part of aging.

More importantly, many forms of arthritis occur in younger individuals.

I have seen patients in their 30s and 40s with inflammatory arthritis that required early and careful treatment.

If we assume all joint pain is due to age, we risk ignoring conditions that need attention.

Why Early Understanding Matters

In the early stages, arthritis may present with mild symptoms.

- Occasional stiffness
- Mild discomfort
- Slight swelling

These may be easy to ignore.

But early understanding makes a difference.

When recognized early:

- Treatment can be started appropriately
- Progression may be slowed
- Long-term damage may be prevented

When ignored:

- Symptoms may worsen
- Joint damage may become permanent
- Treatment becomes more complex

This is why awareness is so important.

Symptoms: The Body's Signals

Your body gives signals when something is not right.

Common symptoms of arthritis include:

- Joint pain
- Morning stiffness
- Swelling
- Warmth around the joint
- Reduced range of movement

- Difficulty with daily activities

The pattern of these symptoms is often more important than their intensity.

A careful observation of these patterns helps guide diagnosis.

Doctor's Pearl

Do not ignore persistent joint symptoms.

A painful joint is not always serious. But a joint that continues to hurt, swell, or stiffen deserves attention.

Early action often leads to better outcomes.

Myth vs Fact

Myth: Arthritis is always due to aging.
Fact: Many types have causes unrelated to age.

Myth: Nothing can be done for arthritis.
Fact: Many effective treatments are available.

Myth: Mild pain means a mild problem.
Fact: Some serious conditions begin with mild symptoms.

CHAPTER 1
ARTHRITIS IS NOT ONE DISEASE

Arthritis is a group of many conditions
that affect the joints in different ways.

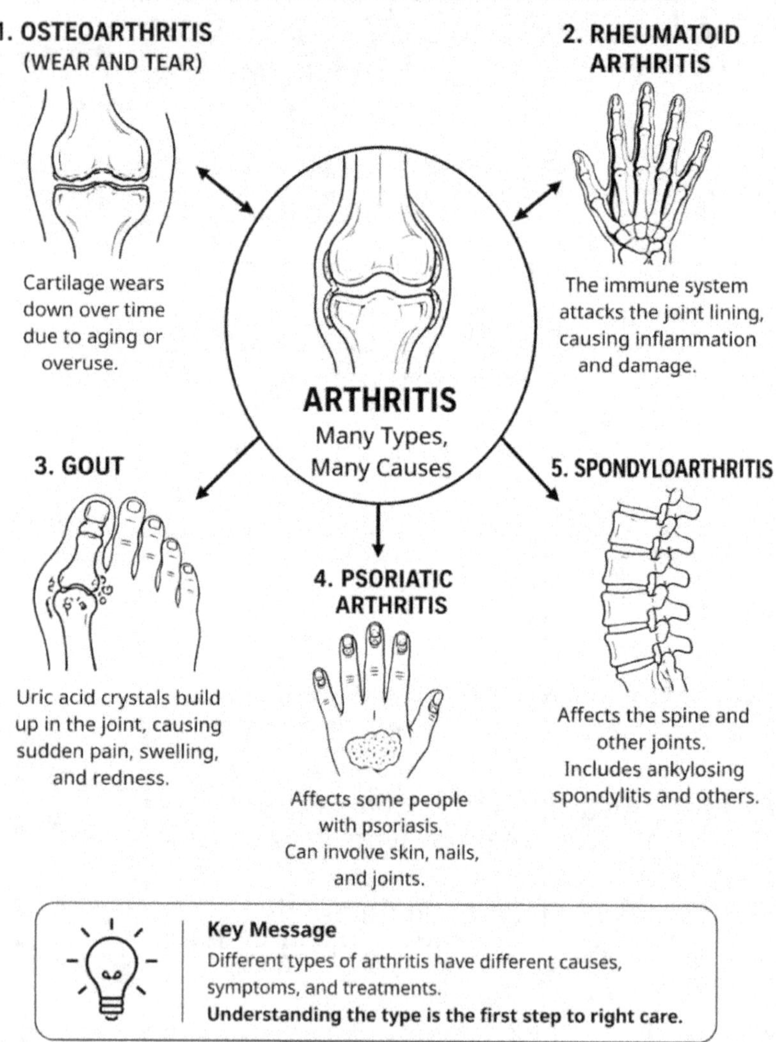

Key Message

Different types of arthritis have different causes,
symptoms, and treatments.
Understanding the type is the first step to right care.

Common Mistakes to Avoid

- Ignoring early symptoms
- Assuming all arthritis is the same
- Self-treating without proper diagnosis
- Avoiding activity completely
- Relying only on temporary pain relief

Red Flag Warnings

Seek medical attention if you notice:

- Sudden severe joint pain with swelling
- Joint pain with fever
- Persistent stiffness lasting more than one hour in the morning
- Rapid loss of joint function
- Inability to bear weight

Key Points

- Arthritis is a group of conditions, not a single disease
- Different types have different causes and treatments
- Early symptoms should not be ignored
- Correct diagnosis is essential

- You can take meaningful steps to manage the condition

Chapter Summary

Arthritis is a broad term that includes many different joint conditions. It can affect people of all ages and may present with pain, stiffness, swelling, and reduced movement. Understanding that arthritis is not a single disease is the first step toward proper diagnosis and effective management.

Action Plan

- Pay attention to persistent joint symptoms
- Observe patterns such as stiffness and swelling
- Avoid self-diagnosis
- Seek timely medical evaluation
- Begin learning about your condition

A Simple Real-Life Example

Two patients came to me with joint pain.

One had knee pain that worsened with activity and improved with rest. The other had swollen fingers with prolonged morning stiffness.

Both said, "I have arthritis."

But their conditions were very different.

One had osteoarthritis. The other had rheumatoid arthritis.

Their treatments were completely different.

That is why understanding the type matters.

Transition to the Next Chapter

Now that you understand what arthritis really means, the next step is to understand the structure it affects.

In the next chapter, we will look inside a **healthy joint** in simple language. Once you understand how a joint normally works, it becomes much easier to understand what goes wrong in arthritis.

CHAPTER 2: How a Healthy Joint Works – Understanding What We Are Trying to Protect

Why This Chapter Is Important

In my experience, something interesting happens when patients understand how a joint works.

They become more careful.
They become more motivated.
And most importantly, they begin to **respect their joints**.

Before we talk about disease, treatment, or prevention, we must understand one simple thing:

What exactly are we trying to protect?

Because when you understand the structure, you understand the problem much better.

A Joint Is Not Just Two Bones

Most people imagine a joint as two bones meeting each other.

That is only a small part of the picture.

A joint is actually a **well-organized system**, where several structures work together smoothly.

These include:

- Bones
- Cartilage
- Synovium (joint lining)
- Synovial fluid
- Ligaments
- Tendons
- Muscles

Each part plays a role. When all parts function well, movement is smooth and painless.

When even one part is affected, the entire system begins to suffer.

Cartilage: The Smooth Cushion

Cartilage is a thin, smooth layer that covers the ends of bones inside a joint.

You never feel it when it is healthy. It works silently.

Its functions are simple but essential:

- It allows bones to glide smoothly
- It reduces friction
- It absorbs shock during movement

Every step you take, every movement you make, depends on this cushion.

But cartilage has one important limitation.

It does not repair easily.

When it begins to wear down, as in osteoarthritis, the joint gradually loses its smooth surface. Friction increases, and pain begins.

Synovium and Joint Fluid: Natural Lubrication

Inside the joint, there is a thin lining called the synovium.

This lining produces synovial fluid.

This fluid:

- Lubricates the joint
- Nourishes the cartilage
- Helps smooth movement

In inflammatory arthritis, this lining becomes irritated and inflamed.

As a result:

- It produces excess fluid
- The joint becomes swollen
- Warmth and pain develop

This is a very different process from simple wear and
tear.

Ligaments: Keeping the Joint Stable

Ligaments connect one bone to another.

They act like strong bands that:

- Hold the joint together
- Maintain stability
- Prevent excessive movement

When ligaments become weak or stretched, the joint
becomes unstable.

This instability increases stress on other parts of the
joint.

Tendons: Connecting Muscle to Bone

Tendons connect muscles to bones.

They allow muscles to move the joint.

Without tendons, even strong muscles cannot produce
movement.

When tendons are irritated or strained:

- Movement becomes painful
- Function is reduced

Tendon problems are often mistaken for joint problems, which can lead to confusion.

Muscles: The Natural Support System

Muscles play a major role in joint health.

Strong muscles:

- Support the joint
- Reduce load on cartilage
- Improve balance and coordination

Weak muscles do the opposite.

They increase stress on the joint and make movement less stable.

This is why strengthening muscles is one of the most important parts of arthritis care.

What Goes Wrong in Arthritis

Different types of arthritis affect different parts of the joint.

- In osteoarthritis, cartilage wears down
- In rheumatoid arthritis, the synovium becomes inflamed
- In gout, crystals deposit inside the joint
- In infection, organisms invade the joint

Even though the causes are different, the end result often looks similar:

- Pain
- Stiffness
- Swelling
- Reduced movement

Understanding which part is affected helps guide treatment.

Why Movement Is Essential

Many patients believe that rest protects a painful joint.

Short rest may help during severe pain.

But complete inactivity causes problems.

Movement:

- Nourishes cartilage
- Maintains flexibility
- Strengthens muscles

- Improves circulation

Without movement:

- Joints become stiff
- Muscles weaken
- Pain increases

The joint is designed to move.

When it stops moving, it begins to deteriorate.

Doctor's Pearl

Joint damage rarely happens suddenly.

It develops slowly, often over years.

If you protect your joints early, you can reduce long-term problems significantly.

Myth vs Fact

Myth: Joints wear out suddenly.
Fact: Most joint damage develops gradually over time.

Myth: Rest is the best treatment for joint pain.
Fact: Controlled movement is essential for joint health.

CHAPTER 2
HOW A HEALTHY JOINT WORKS

A healthy joint allows smooth movement, supports your body, and protects the bones.

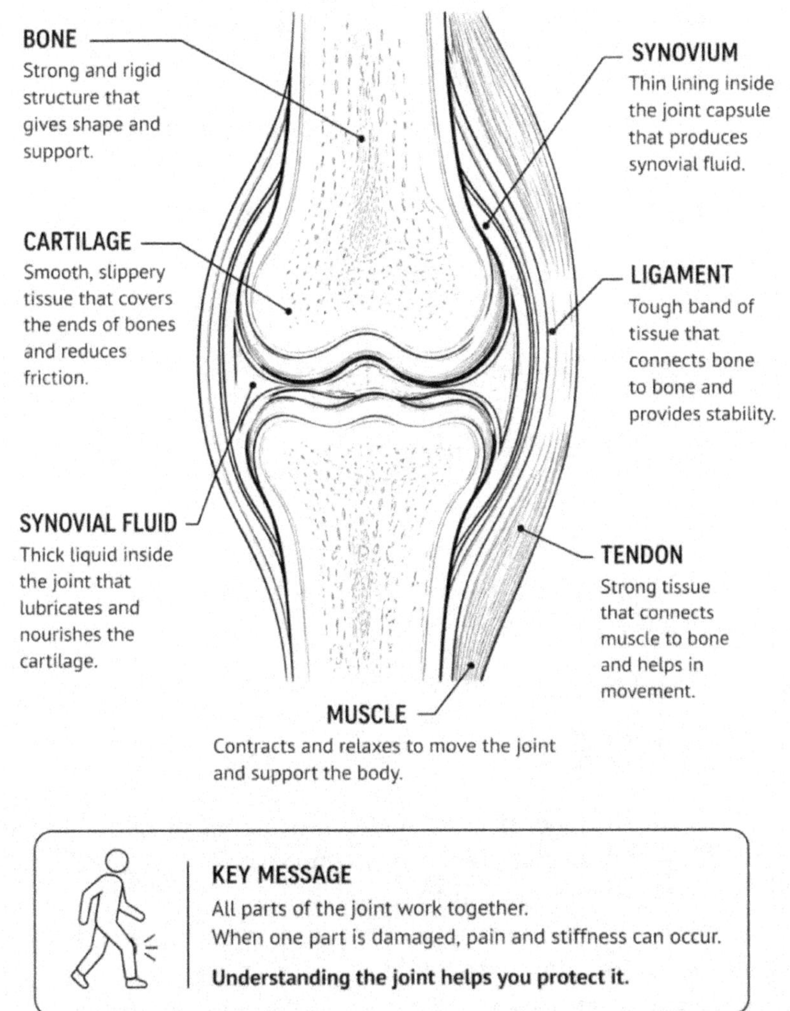

KEY MESSAGE

All parts of the joint work together.
When one part is damaged, pain and stiffness can occur.

Understanding the joint helps you protect it.

Common Mistakes to Avoid

- Ignoring joint health until pain begins
- Avoiding movement due to fear
- Not strengthening muscles
- Poor posture during daily activities
- Repetitive strain without proper technique

Red Flag Warnings

Seek medical attention if you notice:

- Sudden joint swelling
- Severe pain without clear cause
- Rapid loss of movement
- Joint pain with fever
- Persistent symptoms not improving

Key Points

- A joint is a complex system, not just bones
- Cartilage provides smooth movement but has limited repair ability
- Synovial inflammation causes swelling and pain
- Muscles play a key role in joint support
- Movement is essential for joint health

Chapter Summary

A healthy joint depends on the coordinated function of cartilage, synovium, ligaments, tendons, and muscles. Cartilage provides cushioning, synovial fluid lubricates movement, and muscles support stability. Arthritis develops when one or more of these components are affected. Understanding this structure helps you understand how to protect your joints.

Action Plan

- Think of your joints as structures that need care
- Stay physically active with gentle movement
- Begin simple strengthening exercises
- Avoid prolonged inactivity
- Maintain good posture in daily life

A Simple Real-Life Example

A patient once told me, "Doctor, I stopped walking because I thought it would damage my knee."

Over time, his muscles weakened, and his pain worsened.

We started a simple plan with short walks and basic strengthening exercises.

Gradually, his strength improved, and his pain reduced.

He later said, "I did not realize movement would help so much."

That is a lesson worth remembering.

Transition to the Next Chapter

Now that you understand how a healthy joint works, the next step is to understand the different types of arthritis.

In the next chapter, we will clearly explain the **major types of arthritis**, so you can recognize patterns and better understand your own condition.

CHAPTER 3: The Major Types of Arthritis – Understanding What Makes Each One Different

Why This Chapter Matters More Than You Think

When a patient tells me, "Doctor, I have arthritis," I never stop there.

I always ask one more question.

"What type of arthritis?"

Because that single detail changes everything.

Two patients may both have joint pain, stiffness, and swelling. But one may need simple lifestyle measures, while the other may need early, targeted treatment to prevent permanent joint damage.

Same symptom. Very different disease.

This chapter will help you understand the major types of arthritis in a clear, practical way. Once you understand these patterns, you will begin to recognize your own condition more confidently.

A Simple Way to Understand Arthritis Types

To make things easier, I usually group arthritis into three broad categories:

- **Degenerative arthritis** – due to wear and tear
- **Inflammatory arthritis** – due to immune system activity
- **Crystal-related arthritis** – due to deposits in the joint

There are also other types, including infection-related and systemic conditions.

Let us now go through the most important ones you should know.

Osteoarthritis: The Most Common Form

Osteoarthritis is the type most people are referring to when they say they have arthritis.

It develops slowly over time as cartilage wears down.

Common features:

- Pain that worsens with activity
- Stiffness after rest, usually brief
- Gradual progression

- Reduced flexibility

Commonly affected joints:

- Knees
- Hips
- Hands
- Spine

Risk factors:

- Increasing age
- Excess body weight
- Previous joint injury
- Repetitive use of joints

This is the most common type, especially after midlife.

The encouraging part is that many patients improve significantly with **exercise, weight control, and proper guidance**.

Rheumatoid Arthritis: When the Immune System Attacks

Rheumatoid arthritis is very different from osteoarthritis.

Here, the body's immune system attacks the lining of the joints.

Common features:

- Swelling and tenderness
- Morning stiffness lasting more than one hour
- Involvement of both sides of the body
- Fatigue and general discomfort

What makes it important:

- It can damage joints if untreated
- It may lead to deformity
- It can affect other parts of the body

Early diagnosis and treatment are essential to prevent long-term damage.

Gout: Sudden and Severe

Gout is one of the most dramatic forms of arthritis.

It is caused by **uric acid crystals** accumulating in a joint.

Typical features:

- Sudden onset of severe pain
- Often affects the big toe
- Redness, swelling, and warmth
- Extreme tenderness

Patients often say that even the bedsheet touching the joint is painful.

Common triggers:

- Certain foods
- Alcohol
- Dehydration
- Kidney problems

The good news is that gout can be **well controlled and often prevented** with proper treatment.

Psoriatic Arthritis: When Skin and Joints Are Linked

Psoriatic arthritis occurs in people with psoriasis.

Features may include:

- Joint pain with skin lesions
- Swelling of entire fingers or toes
- Nail changes
- Asymmetrical joint involvement

Sometimes joint symptoms appear before skin changes, which can make diagnosis more challenging.

Ankylosing Spondylitis: Involving the Spine

This type mainly affects the spine and nearby joints.

Common features:

- Chronic back pain
- Morning stiffness
- Pain that improves with movement
- Onset at a younger age

This condition behaves differently from common back pain and requires specific management.

Lupus and Other Systemic Conditions

Some diseases affect multiple organs, including joints.

In conditions like lupus:

- Joint pain is common
- There may be fatigue, rash, or other symptoms
- Organs such as kidneys, heart, or lungs may be involved

In these cases, arthritis is part of a **larger systemic illness**.

Infectious Arthritis: A Condition That Needs Urgent Care

Infectious arthritis occurs when bacteria or other organisms enter a joint.

Features include:

- Sudden severe pain
- Swelling and warmth
- Fever
- Rapid progression

This is a medical emergency.

Prompt treatment is essential to prevent permanent damage.

Conditions That Can Mimic Arthritis

Not all joint pain is arthritis.

Other conditions may present similarly:

- Tendon injuries
- Ligament problems
- Bursitis
- Fibromyalgia
- Referred pain from the spine

This is why proper evaluation is important.

Doctor's Pearl

Do not assume all joint pain is the same.

Correct diagnosis is the foundation of effective treatment.

Myth vs Fact

Myth: All arthritis is the same.
Fact: Different types have different causes and treatments.

Myth: What works for one person will work for everyone.
Fact: Treatment must be individualized.

Common Mistakes to Avoid

- Self-diagnosing based on symptoms
- Assuming all arthritis is osteoarthritis
- Ignoring early signs of inflammatory disease
- Delaying proper evaluation
- Using long-term medication without diagnosis

Red Flag Warnings

Seek medical advice if you notice:

- Persistent swelling in multiple joints
- Severe morning stiffness
- Sudden severe pain in one joint
- Joint pain with fever
- Back pain that improves with movement

MAJOR TYPES OF ARTHRITIS

Different types of arthritis have different causes, symptoms, and treatments.

❶ OSTEOARTHRITIS
(WEAR AND TEAR)

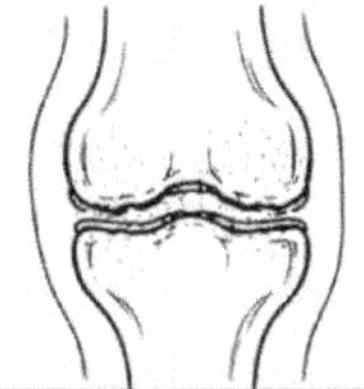

- Caused by wear and tear of cartilage over time.
- Common in older age.
- Affects knees, hips, hands, spine, and other joints.

❷ RHEUMATOID ARTHRITIS
(IMMUNE SYSTEM ATTACK)

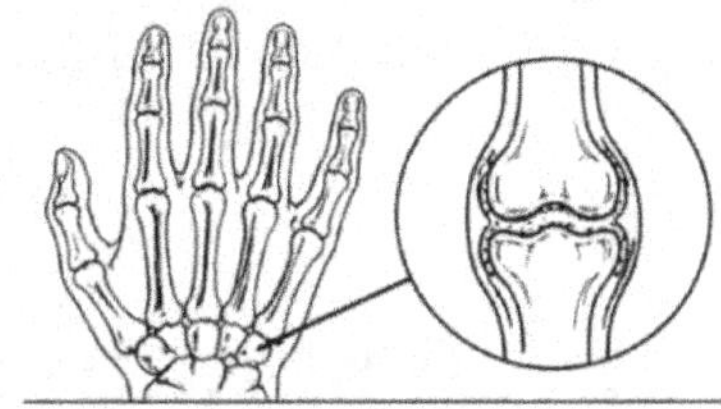

- Caused by the immune system attacking the joint lining.
- Causes inflammation, pain, swelling, and stiffness.
- Can affect many joints.

❸ GOUT ARTHRITIS
(URIC ACID CRYSTALS)

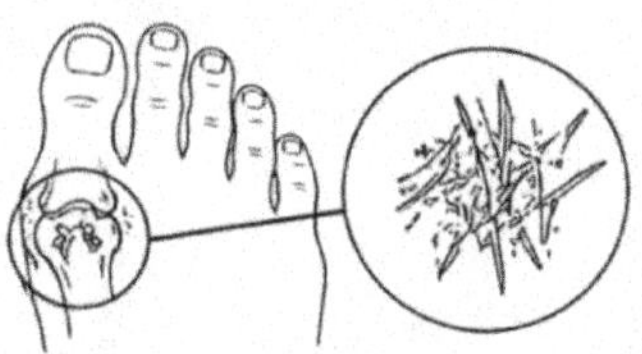

- Caused by buildup of uric acid crystals in the joint.
- Causes sudden, severe pain, redness, and swelling.
- Common in the big toe but can affect other joints.

❹ PSORIATIC ARTHRITIS
(SKIN AND JOINTS)

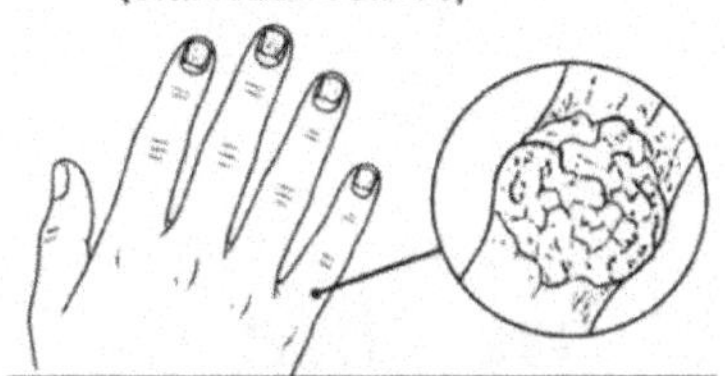

- Affects people with psoriasis.
- Can affect skin, nails, and joints.
- Causes pain, swelling, and stiffness.
- May affect the spine in some people.

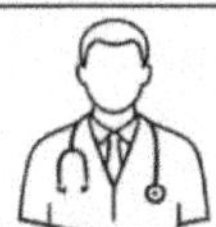

KEY MESSAGE

Knowing the type of arthritis is important for proper treatment and better long-term outcomes.
Early diagnosis and right care make a big difference.

Key Points

- Arthritis includes many different diseases
- Osteoarthritis, rheumatoid arthritis, and gout are the most common
- Some types affect the whole body
- Correct diagnosis is essential
- Early treatment improves outcomes

Chapter Summary

Arthritis is not a single condition but a group of diseases with different causes and patterns. Osteoarthritis is the most common form, while inflammatory and crystal-related types have distinct features and require different treatments. Understanding these differences is the key to effective care.

Action Plan

- Observe your symptoms carefully
- Note which joints are affected
- Track morning stiffness duration
- Avoid self-diagnosis
- Seek proper medical evaluation

A Simple Real-Life Example

Two patients came to me with hand pain.

One had osteoarthritis. His pain worsened with use, and stiffness was brief. He improved with exercise and simple measures.

The other had rheumatoid arthritis. Her stiffness lasted more than an hour, and her joints were swollen. She needed early disease-specific treatment.

Same complaint. Different disease. Different treatment.

Transition to the Next Chapter

Now that you understand the major types of arthritis, the next step is to recognize how these conditions begin.

In the next chapter, we will focus on **early symptoms and warning signs**, so you can identify arthritis at the earliest stage and act in time.

CHAPTER 4: Recognizing Arthritis Early – The Signals Your Body Is Already Giving You

The Quiet Beginning Most People Miss

In my experience, arthritis rarely begins dramatically.

It does not usually announce itself with a sudden, unmistakable event.

Instead, it begins quietly.

A little stiffness in the morning.
A mild ache after activity.
A joint that "does not feel quite right."

Most patients ignore these early signs. Life is busy. The discomfort seems minor. It is easy to assume it will go away.

But here is something I have learned over many years.

Your body almost always gives early warnings.

The difference between patients who do well and those who struggle often comes down to one thing:

Who listens early, and who waits too long.

Joint Pain: Look Beyond the Intensity

Pain is usually the first symptom people notice.

But the intensity of pain is not the most important thing.

The **pattern of pain** tells us much more.

You may notice:

- Pain that increases with activity
- Pain that appears even at rest
- Pain that disturbs sleep
- Sudden, severe pain in a single joint

Each of these patterns gives a clue.

For example:

- Pain with activity often suggests wear and tear
- Pain at rest or at night may suggest inflammation
- Sudden severe pain in one joint may suggest gout or infection

Pain is not random. It is information.

Morning Stiffness: One of the Most Valuable Clues

If there is one symptom I pay special attention to, it is **morning stiffness**.

Patients often describe it in simple words:

"Doctor, my joints feel tight when I wake up."
"It takes time before I can move normally."

The **duration** of stiffness is very important:

- A few minutes suggests a mechanical problem like osteoarthritis
- More than one hour suggests inflammatory arthritis

This simple observation can guide diagnosis more than many tests.

Swelling, Warmth, and Redness

When a joint becomes swollen, it is asking for attention.

You may notice:

- Puffiness around the joint
- Warmth compared to nearby areas
- Redness in some cases
- A feeling of fullness or tightness

Swelling usually indicates inflammation.

It should not be ignored, especially if it persists or recurs.

CHAPTER 4
EARLY WARNING SIGNS OF ARTHRITIS

Recognizing early signs helps in early diagnosis
and better treatment.

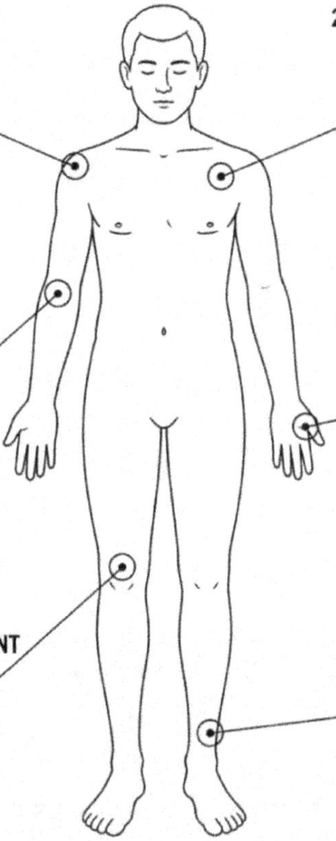

1. JOINT PAIN

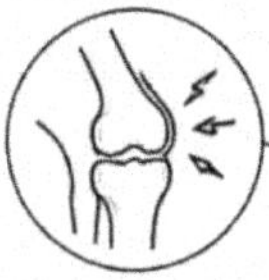

Persistent pain in one
or more joints, which
may get worse with
activity or at rest.

2. MORNING STIFFNESS

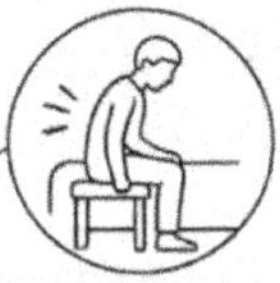

Stiffness in the joints
after waking up,
usually lasting more
than 30 minutes.

3. SWELLING

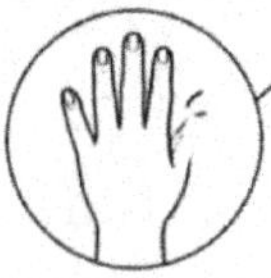

Swelling around
the joints due to
inflammation or
fluid buildup.

4. WARMTH

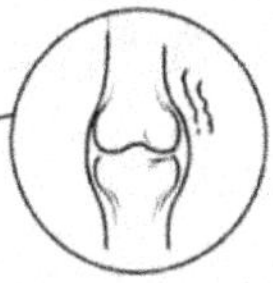

The joint may feel
warm and look red
due to inflammation.

5. REDUCED MOVEMENT

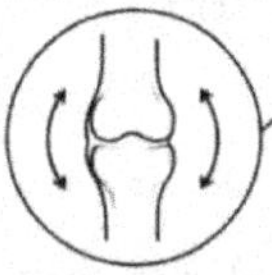

Difficulty in moving
the joint fully.
Stiffness or blockage
during movement.

6. FATIGUE

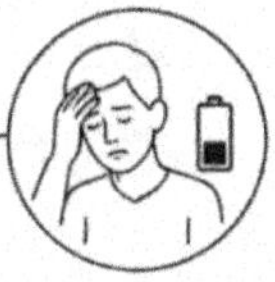

Feeling tired or low
in energy, which is
common in many
types of arthritis.

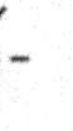

KEY MESSAGE

If you notice any of these signs for more than a few days,
do not ignore them. Consult your doctor early.
Early action can prevent joint damage and improve quality of life.

Loss of Movement: The Slow Change

One of the most overlooked symptoms is gradual loss of movement.

It happens slowly, and many patients adjust without realizing it.

You may notice:

- Difficulty bending or straightening a joint
- Trouble gripping objects
- Reduced walking distance
- Difficulty getting up from a chair

These changes may seem small at first, but over time they affect independence.

Fatigue: The Symptom That Surprises Patients

Many patients are surprised when I ask about fatigue.

They say, "Doctor, I feel tired all the time, but I thought it was just age."

In some types of arthritis, especially inflammatory ones, fatigue is common.

This is not normal tiredness.

It may feel like:

- Low energy despite rest
- Difficulty concentrating
- A general sense of being unwell

This symptom deserves attention.

Symmetry: A Useful Pattern

Another important clue is whether symptoms appear on one side or both.

- **Symmetrical involvement** (both hands, both knees) often suggests inflammatory arthritis
- **Asymmetrical involvement** may suggest osteoarthritis or other conditions

Patterns matter.

They help connect symptoms to the underlying cause.

Flare-Ups: When Symptoms Come and Go

Many types of arthritis do not follow a steady pattern.

Instead, symptoms may come and go.

During a flare, you may notice:

- Increased pain
- More stiffness
- Swelling
- Reduced movement

Then symptoms improve again.

This pattern can be confusing, but it is common.

Recognizing your flares helps you manage them better.

Doctor's Pearl

One symptom alone may not mean much.

But a pattern of symptoms, especially when repeated over time, often tells a clear story.

Myth vs Fact

Myth: If pain comes and goes, it is not serious.
Fact: Many types of arthritis present with flare-ups in early stages.

Myth: Only severe pain needs medical attention.
Fact: Mild but persistent symptoms can indicate early disease.

Common Mistakes to Avoid

- Ignoring mild but recurring symptoms
- Assuming all pain is due to aging
- Waiting until symptoms become severe
- Not paying attention to morning stiffness
- Using repeated pain relief without evaluation

Red Flag Warnings

Seek medical attention if you notice:

- Sudden severe joint pain with swelling
- Joint pain with fever
- Morning stiffness lasting more than one hour
- Rapid loss of movement
- Inability to use or bear weight on a joint

Key Points

- Early symptoms are often subtle
- Pain pattern provides important clues
- Morning stiffness is highly significant
- Swelling suggests inflammation
- Early recognition improves outcomes

Chapter Summary

Arthritis often begins with subtle symptoms such as mild pain, stiffness, or swelling. The pattern of these symptoms, including morning stiffness, symmetry, and flare-ups, provides important clues to the underlying condition. Recognizing these early signals allows timely diagnosis and better long-term outcomes.

Action Plan

- Pay attention to any persistent joint symptoms
- Observe how long morning stiffness lasts
- Notice swelling, warmth, or redness
- Track patterns over time
- Seek medical advice early

A Simple Real-Life Example

A patient came to me with mild stiffness in her fingers every morning.

She had ignored it for several months, thinking it was due to overuse.

On evaluation, she was found to have early rheumatoid arthritis.

Because treatment started early, her condition remained well controlled.

Had she waited longer, the outcome could have been very different.

Transition to the Next Chapter

Now that you understand how arthritis begins and how to recognize early symptoms, the next step is to understand where these symptoms appear.

In the next chapter, we will look at **arthritis in different joints**, helping you connect your symptoms to specific areas of the body.

CHAPTER 5: Arthritis in Different Joints – Understanding the Pattern of Pain

Why Location Tells a Story

When a patient says, "Doctor, my joints hurt," I always ask one more question:

"Which joints?"

That answer often brings us very close to the diagnosis.

Arthritis does not affect the body randomly. Different types tend to involve specific joints and follow recognizable patterns.

If you learn to observe **where the pain is and how it behaves**, you begin to understand your condition much more clearly.

The Knee: The Most Commonly Affected Joint

The knee carries your body weight every day. It works hard, and over time, it is often the first joint to show problems.

Common symptoms:

- Pain while walking or climbing stairs
- Difficulty getting up from a chair
- Stiffness after sitting
- Swelling after activity
- A grinding or cracking sensation

This pattern is very common in osteoarthritis.

Over time, untreated knee arthritis can reduce mobility and confidence in walking. But with proper care, many patients improve significantly.

The Hip: Pain That Is Often Misleading

Hip arthritis can be difficult to recognize because the pain is not always where you expect it.

You may feel:

- Pain in the groin
- Discomfort in the thigh
- Pain that seems to come from the knee
- Difficulty putting on shoes or socks
- Stiffness when getting up

Because of this pattern, hip arthritis is sometimes mistaken for a muscle or back problem.

Recognizing it early helps avoid delay in treatment.

CHAPTER 5
ARTHRITIS IN DIFFERENT JOINTS

Arthritis can affect any joint in the body.
Common joints and typical symptoms are shown below.

1. HANDS & FINGERS

- Pain, swelling, and stiffness in the small joints.
- Difficulty in gripping, writing, or using hands.

2. ELBOWS

- Pain or stiffness.
- Hard to straighten or bend fully.

3. HIPS

- Deep pain in the groin, hip, or buttock.
- Stiffness and difficulty in walking or climbing.

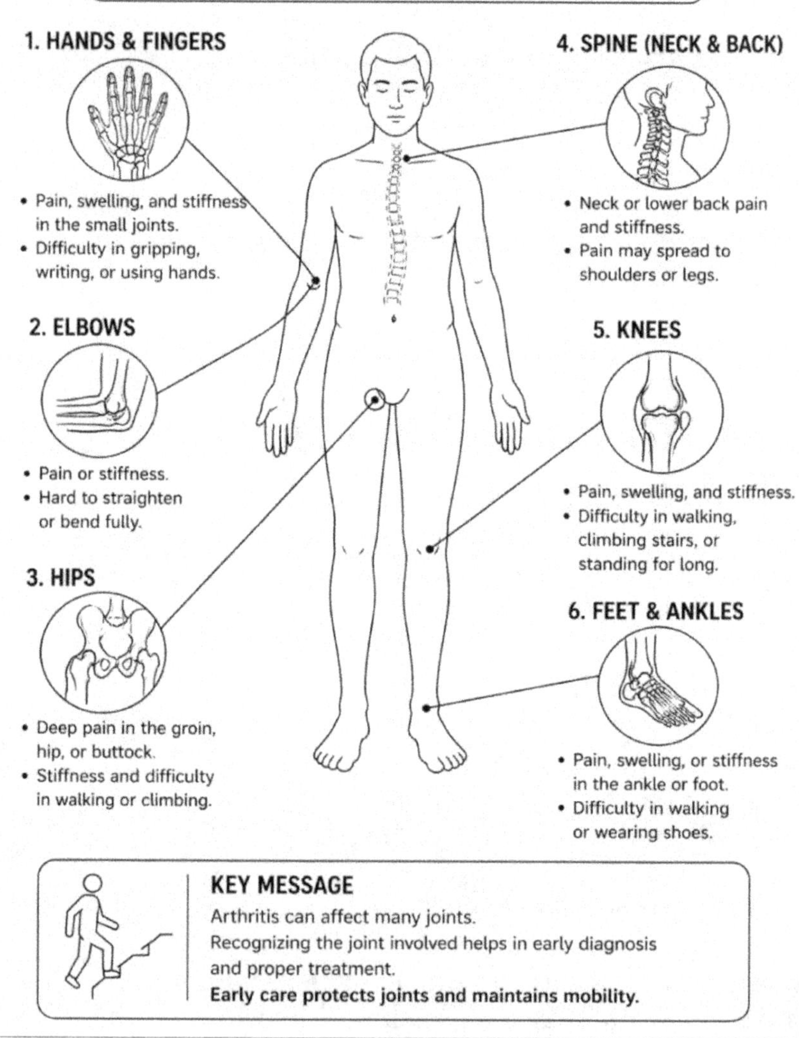

4. SPINE (NECK & BACK)

- Neck or lower back pain and stiffness.
- Pain may spread to shoulders or legs.

5. KNEES

- Pain, swelling, and stiffness.
- Difficulty in walking, climbing stairs, or standing for long.

6. FEET & ANKLES

- Pain, swelling, or stiffness in the ankle or foot.
- Difficulty in walking or wearing shoes.

KEY MESSAGE

Arthritis can affect many joints.
Recognizing the joint involved helps in early diagnosis and proper treatment.
Early care protects joints and maintains mobility.

Hands and Fingers: Small Joints, Big Impact

The hands are involved in almost every daily activity.

Even mild arthritis here can affect independence.

Common symptoms:

- Pain while gripping or pinching
- Morning stiffness
- Swelling of small joints
- Difficulty opening jars or turning keys

In osteoarthritis, joints may develop firm, bony enlargements.

In inflammatory arthritis, swelling may be softer and involve multiple joints on both sides.

Early recognition is important.

The Spine and Neck: More Than Just Back Pain

Arthritis can affect the spine and neck.

You may notice:

- Neck stiffness
- Reduced movement

- Lower back pain
- Pain that travels to arms or legs
- Morning stiffness that improves with movement

In some conditions, especially inflammatory ones, back pain improves with activity and worsens with rest.

This is different from common mechanical back pain.

Feet and Ankles: Often Overlooked

Foot and ankle symptoms are frequently ignored or blamed on footwear.

But arthritis here can cause:

- Pain while walking or standing
- Swelling around the ankle
- Changes in walking pattern
- Difficulty maintaining balance

In gout, the big toe is a classic site of sudden severe pain.

Your feet carry your entire body weight. Their health is essential.

Shoulders and Elbows: Limiting Reach and Strength

These joints may not be affected as commonly as knees or hands, but when they are, daily life is affected.

Symptoms include:

- Pain while lifting the arm
- Difficulty reaching overhead
- Reduced range of motion
- Weakness

Simple tasks like combing hair or lifting objects may become difficult.

One Joint or Many: A Key Difference

The number of joints involved provides an important clue.

- **One joint (monoarthritis):** think of gout, infection, or injury
- **Multiple joints (polyarthritis):** think of inflammatory arthritis

This simple distinction helps guide evaluation.

Doctor's Pearl

Always connect **location with pattern**.

A painful knee alone tells one story.
Pain in both hands with long morning stiffness tells
another.

The more clearly you observe, the better your doctor can
help you.

Myth vs Fact

Myth: Pain in one joint is not serious.
Fact: Sudden severe pain in one joint may require urgent
attention.

Myth: Back pain is always due to strain.
Fact: Some types of arthritis affect the spine.

Common Mistakes to Avoid

- Ignoring early hand symptoms
- Assuming all back pain is mechanical
- Missing hip arthritis that presents as knee pain
- Neglecting foot pain
- Not reporting multiple joint involvement

Red Flag Warnings

Seek medical advice if you notice:

- Sudden severe swelling in a joint
- Persistent back stiffness, especially in the morning
- Rapid loss of joint movement
- Difficulty walking
- Pain that does not improve with rest

Key Points

- Different types of arthritis affect different joints
- Knees, hips, hands, and spine are commonly involved
- Location and pattern together guide diagnosis
- Small joint symptoms can have a large impact
- Early attention prevents long-term problems

Chapter Summary

Arthritis affects different joints in characteristic patterns. Knee arthritis is common and often linked to wear and tear. Hip arthritis may present as groin or thigh pain. Hand arthritis affects daily function, and spine involvement may present as chronic stiffness. Recognizing these patterns helps in early diagnosis and proper management.

Action Plan

- Identify which joints are affected

- Observe whether symptoms are on one side or both
- Note difficulties in daily activities
- Do not ignore small joint symptoms
- Seek evaluation if symptoms persist

A Simple Real-Life Example

A patient came with knee pain and was being treated for osteoarthritis.

On careful questioning, he also had morning stiffness in both hands. Examination showed swelling in small joints.

He was diagnosed with rheumatoid arthritis, and his treatment changed completely.

His symptoms improved significantly.

The lesson is simple.

Do not focus on just one joint. See the whole pattern.

Transition to the Next Chapter

Now that you understand how arthritis affects different joints, the next step is to look beyond the joints.

In the next chapter, we will explore how arthritis can affect **energy, sleep, mood, and overall health**, and why treating the whole person matters.

CHAPTER 6: Arthritis Beyond the Joints – Understanding the Whole-Body Impact

Looking at the Bigger Picture

When most people think about arthritis, they picture a painful knee or a stiff hand.

But in real life, arthritis rarely stays limited to one joint.

Over time, it begins to influence how you move, how you sleep, how you feel, and even how you think about your health.

In my practice, I have seen this again and again.

If we focus only on the joint, we miss the full picture.

To manage arthritis properly, we must understand its effect on the entire body.

Mobility and Independence: The First Changes

The earliest impact of arthritis is usually on movement.

You may notice:

- Slower walking
- Difficulty climbing stairs
- Trouble getting up from a chair
- Reduced ability to lift or carry

At first, these changes are subtle. Many patients adjust quietly.

They avoid certain movements. They take shortcuts. They ask for help more often.

Over time, this can affect **independence**, which is one of the most important aspects of quality of life.

Muscle Weakness: The Hidden Problem

Pain changes behavior.

When joints hurt, people naturally move less.

But reduced movement leads to:

- Weak muscles
- Less joint support
- Increased stress on joints
- More pain

This creates a cycle:

Less movement → weaker muscles → more joint stress → more pain → even less movement

Breaking this cycle is essential.

Fatigue: More Than Just Tiredness

Many patients say, "Doctor, I feel tired all the time."

This fatigue is not the same as normal tiredness.

It may feel like:

- Low energy even after rest
- Difficulty concentrating
- A general sense of heaviness

Fatigue may be caused by:

- Chronic inflammation
- Poor sleep due to pain
- Reduced physical activity
- Emotional stress

It is a real symptom and should not be ignored.

Sleep Disturbance: The Pain–Sleep Cycle

Pain and sleep are closely connected.

- Pain makes it difficult to fall asleep
- Discomfort causes frequent waking
- Poor sleep increases pain sensitivity

This creates a cycle:

Pain leads to poor sleep, and poor sleep increases pain.

Improving sleep often improves pain as well.

Emotional Health: An Important Part of Care

Living with a long-term condition is not easy.

Over time, arthritis can affect emotional well-being.

You may feel:

- Frustration
- Worry about the future
- Reduced confidence
- Low mood

These feelings are natural.

Ignoring them makes management more difficult. Addressing them improves overall outcomes.

ARTHRITIS AFFECTS THE WHOLE BODY

Arthritis is not just a joint problem.
It can affect many parts of your body and life.

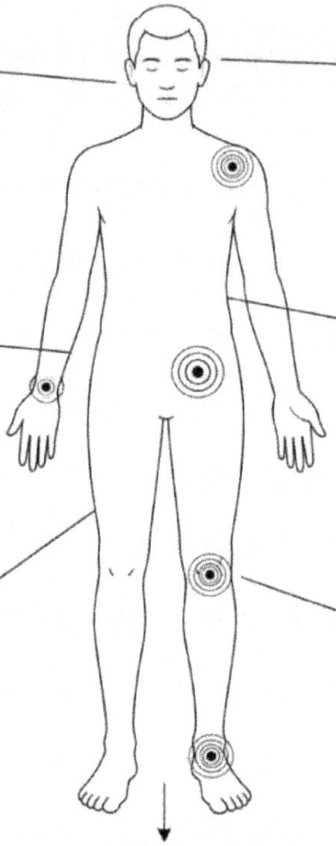

1. POOR SLEEP

Pain and stiffness can disturb sleep, leading to tiredness and low energy.

2. MOOD CHANGES

Chronic pain and limitations can cause stress, anxiety, and depression.

3. FATIGUE

Ongoing inflammation and pain can make you feel constantly tired.

4. HEART HEALTH

Some types of arthritis increase the risk of heart disease and other problems.

5. WEIGHT GAIN

Less activity and pain can lead to weight gain, which puts more stress on joints.

6. REDUCED MOBILITY

Joint pain and stiffness can make daily activities difficult and reduce independence.

7. IMPACT ON DAILY LIFE

Work Productivity

Family & Social Life

Hobbies & Leisure

Financial Stress

KEY MESSAGE

Arthritis affects more than joints. It can impact your body, mind, and daily life.
Managing arthritis is about caring for your overall health.

Effects on the Heart and Metabolism

This is something many patients are not aware of.

Inflammatory arthritis, especially conditions like rheumatoid arthritis, is associated with increased risk of:

- Heart disease
- High blood pressure
- Metabolic problems

Chronic inflammation affects the entire body, including blood vessels.

Even in non-inflammatory arthritis, reduced activity and weight gain may indirectly increase these risks.

Effects on Other Organs

Some types of arthritis are part of systemic conditions.

For example:

- Rheumatoid arthritis may affect lungs and eyes
- Lupus may affect kidneys, heart, and brain
- Psoriatic arthritis affects skin and nails

In these conditions, arthritis is only one part of a broader disease.

Impact on Daily Life

Arthritis affects how you live your life.

You may notice:

- Reduced work efficiency
- Difficulty participating in social activities
- Changes in family roles
- Increased dependence

Patients often say, "I cannot do what I used to do."

Understanding this impact helps us manage the condition better.

Doctor's Pearl

Treat the whole person, not just the joint.

When we address movement, sleep, emotional health, and lifestyle together, outcomes are much better.

Myth vs Fact

Myth: Arthritis only affects joints.
Fact: It can affect energy, sleep, mood, and overall health.

Myth: Fatigue is unrelated to arthritis.
Fact: Fatigue is a common symptom, especially in inflammatory conditions.

Common Mistakes to Avoid

- Ignoring fatigue and sleep problems
- Avoiding activity completely
- Focusing only on pain
- Neglecting emotional health
- Delaying lifestyle changes

Red Flag Warnings

Seek medical advice if you notice:

- Severe or persistent fatigue
- Ongoing sleep problems
- Symptoms of depression or anxiety
- Rapid decline in daily function
- New or unexplained symptoms

Key Points

- Arthritis affects the whole body
- Mobility and independence may decline
- Muscle weakness worsens joint problems
- Fatigue and sleep disturbances are common

- Emotional health is important

Chapter Summary

Arthritis is not just a joint problem. It affects movement, muscle strength, energy, sleep, emotional health, and overall well-being. Inflammatory types can also increase the risk of cardiovascular disease and affect other organs. Effective management requires a comprehensive, whole-body approach.

Action Plan

- Stay physically active within your limits
- Begin gentle strengthening exercises
- Improve sleep habits
- Address fatigue and emotional health
- Maintain regular medical follow-up
- Focus on overall well-being, not just joint pain

A Simple Real-Life Example

A patient once told me, "Doctor, my pain is manageable, but I feel exhausted all the time."

We worked on improving sleep, increasing gentle activity, and managing stress.

Within weeks, his energy improved significantly.

His pain had not changed much, but his quality of life improved greatly.

That is an important lesson.

Transition to the Next Chapter

Now that you understand how arthritis affects the whole body, the next step is to understand what happens if it is not properly managed.

In the next chapter, we will discuss the **complications of untreated arthritis** and why early care is so important.

CHAPTER 7: Complications of Untreated Arthritis – What Happens If We Wait Too Long

An Honest Conversation

From time to time, a patient looks at me and says,

"Doctor, the pain is there, but I can manage. Do I really need to do anything more?"

It is an honest question. And it deserves an honest answer.

Arthritis is often slow. It does not always force you to act immediately. That is exactly why many people delay treatment.

But here is the truth.

Slow does not mean harmless.

Over time, untreated or poorly controlled arthritis can lead to damage that cannot be reversed. The goal of treatment is not only to reduce pain today, but to protect your joints and your independence for the future.

CHAPTER 7
WHAT HAPPENS IF ARTHRITIS IS IGNORED

Ignoring arthritis can lead to worsening symptoms, joint damage, and loss of independence.

 **EARLY PAIN AND STIFFNESS**

 **INCREASED INFLAMMATION AND SWELLING**

 **JOINT DAMAGE BEGINS**

 **LOSS OF MOVEMENT AND FUNCTION**

 **LOSS OF INDEPENDENCE AND QUALITY OF LIFE**

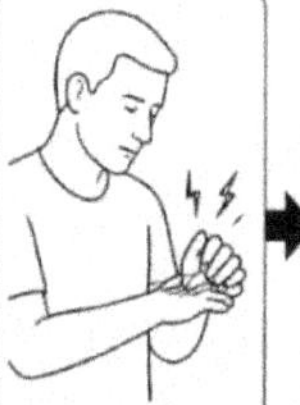
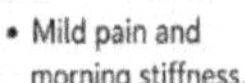

- Mild pain and morning stiffness.
- Symptoms come and go.
- May be ignored or considered normal.

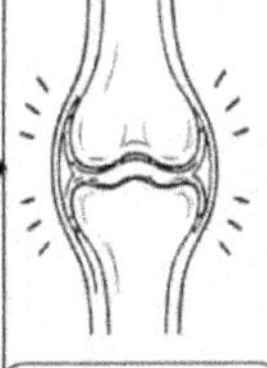

- Pain becomes more frequent.
- Swelling, warmth, and tenderness develop.
- Daily activities start becoming difficult.

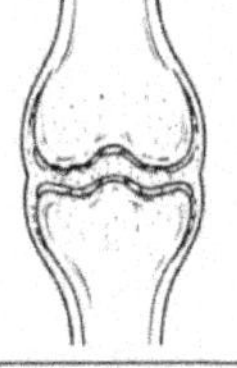

- Cartilage wears away.
- Bone damage may start.
- Stiffness and pain increase.

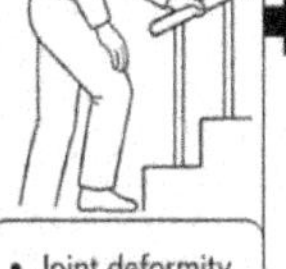

- Joint deformity may develop.
- Movement becomes limited.
- Difficulty in walking, bending, and performing daily tasks.

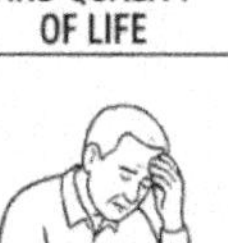

- Need help for daily activities.
- Reduced independence.
- Poor quality of life and emotional impact.

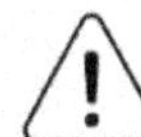

IMPORTANT

Early diagnosis and proper treatment can slow down or prevent these changes and help you live an active and independent life.

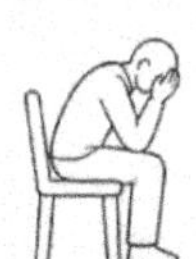

IGNORE TODAY

More pain, more damage, more disability, less independence.

VS

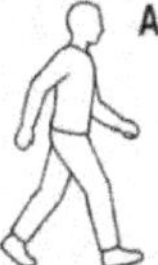

ACT EARLY

Less pain, less damage, better function, more independence and a better life.

KEY MESSAGE

Do not wait and watch. Early action protects your joints, preserves your function, and improves your future.
Your joints will thank you for the care you give today.

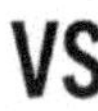

Progressive Joint Damage: A Silent Process

One of the most important consequences of untreated arthritis is gradual joint damage.

This process may include:

- Thinning of cartilage
- Narrowing of joint space
- Increased friction between bones
- Weakening of supporting structures

In inflammatory arthritis, this damage may occur even faster because the immune system continues to attack the joint.

The problem is that this damage develops quietly.

By the time it becomes obvious, it may already be advanced.

Chronic Pain: Harder to Control Over Time

Early arthritis pain may be occasional.

With time, untreated disease can lead to:

- Persistent pain
- Pain at rest

- Pain that interferes with sleep
- Increased sensitivity to pain

Chronic pain is not just physical. It also affects the nervous system and emotional well-being.

Managing long-standing pain is often more difficult than controlling it early.

Loss of Movement and Function

As joints become more damaged, movement becomes restricted.

You may begin to notice:

- Reduced walking distance
- Difficulty climbing stairs
- Trouble with daily activities
- Slower movements

Many patients gradually adjust their lifestyle to cope.

But over time, this can lead to **loss of independence**, which has a significant impact on quality of life.

Muscle Weakness and Instability

Pain leads to less movement.

Less movement leads to weaker muscles.

Weak muscles:

- Provide less support to joints
- Increase stress on damaged areas
- Reduce balance and coordination

This increases the risk of further joint damage and instability.

Bone Loss and Fracture Risk

Chronic inflammation and inactivity can weaken bones.

In addition:

- Long-term use of certain medications, especially steroids, may reduce bone strength
- Reduced physical activity leads to decreased bone density

This increases the risk of osteoporosis and fractures.

Increased Risk of Falls

Stiff joints and weak muscles affect balance.

You may experience:

- Unsteady walking
- Slower reaction time
- Difficulty correcting posture

These changes increase the risk of falls, which can lead to serious injuries.

Effects on the Heart and Overall Health

This is an important but often overlooked aspect.

Inflammatory arthritis is associated with increased risk of:

- Heart disease
- Stroke
- High blood pressure

Chronic inflammation affects blood vessels and overall health.

Even in osteoarthritis, reduced activity and weight gain can indirectly increase these risks.

Effects on Other Organs

Some types of arthritis are part of systemic diseases.

For example:

- Rheumatoid arthritis may affect lungs and eyes
- Lupus may affect kidneys, heart, and brain
- Psoriatic arthritis may involve skin and nails

Ignoring these conditions can lead to complications beyond the joints.

Problems Related to Medication Misuse

Another risk comes from improper treatment.

- Long-term unsupervised use of pain medicines can affect the stomach, kidneys, and heart
- Excessive use of steroids can lead to weight gain, diabetes, and bone loss

This is why proper guidance is essential.

Doctor's Pearl

The goal is not just to relieve pain.

It is to **prevent damage before it becomes permanent**.

Myth vs Fact

Myth: Arthritis is slow, so treatment can wait.
Fact: Even slow diseases can cause permanent damage over time.

Myth: If pain is tolerable, the condition is under control.
Fact: Damage may continue even when pain seems mild.

Common Mistakes to Avoid

- Ignoring persistent symptoms
- Delaying medical evaluation
- Using long-term pain relief without diagnosis
- Avoiding activity completely
- Not following treatment plans

Red Flag Warnings

Seek medical advice if you notice:

- Rapid worsening of symptoms
- Visible changes in joint shape
- Severe limitation of movement
- Frequent falls
- Symptoms involving other organs

Key Points

- Untreated arthritis can cause permanent joint damage
- Chronic pain becomes harder to manage over time
- Mobility and independence may decline
- Inflammatory arthritis can affect other organs
- Early treatment improves outcomes

Chapter Summary

If arthritis is not properly managed, it can lead to progressive joint damage, chronic pain, reduced mobility, and loss of independence. Inflammatory types may also affect the heart and other organs. Early diagnosis and consistent treatment are essential to prevent these complications.

Action Plan

- Do not ignore persistent joint symptoms
- Seek early medical evaluation
- Follow treatment plans consistently
- Stay physically active within your limits
- Monitor for new or worsening symptoms
- Maintain regular follow-up

A Simple Real-Life Example

Two patients came to me with early symptoms.

One chose to wait, hoping the problem would improve on its own. Over time, his joints became damaged, and his mobility declined.

The other started treatment early and followed a structured plan. Years later, she remains active and independent.

The difference was not the disease.

The difference was **timing and consistency**.

Transition to the Next Chapter

Now that you understand the risks of untreated arthritis, the next step is to understand how we make the correct diagnosis.

In the next chapter, we will walk through the **step-by-step process of diagnosing arthritis**, so you can understand how decisions are made and avoid confusion.

CHAPTER 8: How Arthritis Is Diagnosed – Finding the Right Answer with Clarity

Why Diagnosis Changes Everything

In many patients, there is a turning point.

Before that point, there is confusion.

Pain is treated on and off. Different remedies are tried. Advice comes from multiple sources. Nothing feels certain.

Then comes the correct diagnosis.

And suddenly, things begin to make sense.

Treatment becomes focused. Decisions become clearer. Anxiety reduces.

That is why diagnosis is not just a label.
It is the **foundation of proper care**.

Diagnosis Is Not One Test

Many patients come with reports in hand and ask,

"Doctor, what does this test show? Do I have arthritis?"

It is a very natural question.

But here is the important point.

No single test can diagnose all types of arthritis.

Diagnosis is a combination of:

- Your symptoms
- Your medical history
- Physical examination
- Selected tests

Each part adds a piece to the puzzle.

Step 1: Your Story – The Most Valuable Clue

The most important step in diagnosis is listening carefully to your symptoms.

You may be asked:

- When did the pain begin?
- Which joints are involved?
- Is the pain worse with activity or at rest?
- How long does morning stiffness last?
- Do symptoms come and go?
- Is there swelling, warmth, or redness?
- Do you feel fatigue or general discomfort?

These details are extremely important.

In many cases, a careful history alone gives a strong indication of the type of arthritis.

Step 2: Physical Examination – What We Can See and Feel

After listening to your history, the next step is examination.

Your doctor may assess:

- Swelling of joints
- Tenderness
- Warmth
- Range of movement
- Muscle strength
- Walking pattern

Patterns again become important.

For example:

- Symmetrical swelling in small joints suggests inflammatory arthritis
- Limited movement with bony enlargement suggests osteoarthritis

Examination confirms and refines the diagnosis.

CHAPTER 8
HOW ARTHRITIS IS DIAGNOSED

A proper diagnosis is the first step
toward the right treatment and better outcomes.

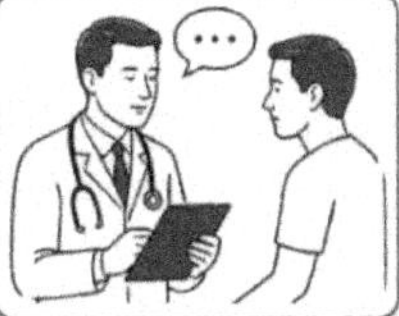

① MEDICAL HISTORY AND SYMPTOMS

Your doctor asks about your pain, stiffness, other symptoms, and medical history.

- When did symptoms start?
- Which joints are affected?
- Morning stiffness?
- Family history?
- Other medical conditions?

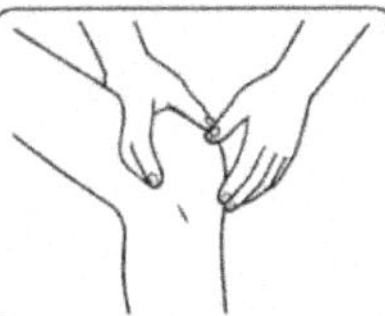

② PHYSICAL EXAMINATION

Your doctor examines your joints, muscles, and overall movement.

- Check for swelling, warmth, or redness
- Check range of motion
- Check for tenderness
- Check other body systems

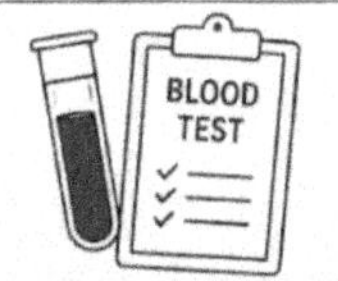

③ BLOOD TESTS

Blood tests help identify inflammation, autoimmunity, or other underlying problems.

- ESR, CRP (inflammation)
- Rheumatoid factor (RF)
- Anti-CCP antibody
- Uric acid level
- Others as needed

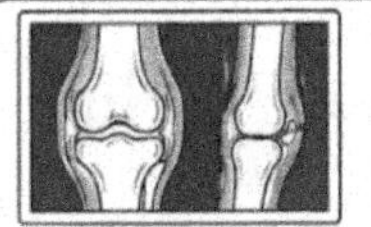

④ IMAGING TESTS

Imaging helps look at the joint structures in detail.

- X-rays
- Ultrasound
- MRI (if needed)
- CT scan (if needed)

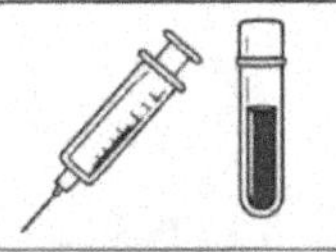

⑤ JOINT FLUID ANALYSIS

If there is swelling, fluid may be taken from the joint and tested.

- Check for infection
- Check for crystals (gout)
- Check for inflammation
- Helps in accurate diagnosis

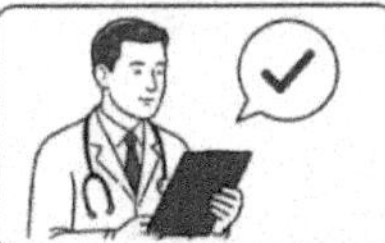

⑥ DIAGNOSIS AND PLAN

All findings are combined to reach a diagnosis and create a treatment plan.

- Confirm the type of arthritis
- Assess severity
- Plan the right treatment
- Discuss goals and follow-up

KEY MESSAGE

A careful evaluation helps identify the correct type of arthritis.
This leads to the right treatment, less pain, and better long-term results.
Do not self-diagnose. Consult your doctor for proper diagnosis.

Step 3: Blood Tests – Helpful but Not Definitive

Blood tests are useful, but they must be interpreted carefully.

Common tests include:

- ESR and CRP – markers of inflammation
- Rheumatoid factor (RF)
- Anti-CCP antibodies
- ANA for autoimmune diseases
- Uric acid levels for gout

It is important to remember:

- Normal results do not always rule out disease
- Abnormal results do not always confirm disease

Tests support the diagnosis. They do not replace clinical judgment.

Step 4: Imaging – Seeing Inside the Joint

Imaging helps us understand structural changes.

X-rays

- Show joint space narrowing and bone changes
- Useful in osteoarthritis and advanced disease

Ultrasound

- Detects inflammation and fluid
- Useful in early inflammatory conditions

MRI

- Provides detailed images
- Detects early changes not visible on X-rays

Not every patient needs every test. The choice depends on the clinical situation.

Step 5: Joint Fluid Analysis – When Needed

In certain cases, especially when a joint is swollen, fluid may be removed for testing.

This is called joint aspiration.

It helps to:

- Detect infection
- Identify uric acid crystals in gout
- Differentiate between types of arthritis

This is a very valuable test in the right situation.

Why Diagnosis May Take Time

Sometimes diagnosis is not immediately clear.

This can happen because:

- Early disease may not show clear signs
- Tests may be normal in early stages
- Symptoms may overlap

In such cases, follow-up becomes important.

With time, the pattern becomes clearer.

Doctor's Pearl

Treat the patient, not just the report.

I have seen patients with abnormal tests but no significant disease. I have also seen patients with normal tests but clear arthritis based on symptoms and examination.

The full picture always matters.

Myth vs Fact

Myth: A blood test alone can diagnose arthritis.
Fact: Diagnosis requires a complete clinical evaluation.

Myth: Normal test results mean nothing is wrong.
Fact: Early arthritis may not show abnormalities.

Common Mistakes to Avoid

- Relying only on lab reports
- Ignoring symptoms
- Self-diagnosing based on tests
- Repeating unnecessary investigations
- Delaying proper evaluation

Red Flag Warnings

Seek medical attention if you notice:

- Sudden severe joint swelling
- Joint pain with fever
- Rapid worsening of symptoms
- Loss of joint function
- Signs of infection

Key Points

- Diagnosis is a step-by-step process
- History and examination are most important
- Tests support but do not replace clinical judgment
- Imaging helps assess joint structure
- Follow-up may be needed for clarity

Chapter Summary

Diagnosing arthritis involves careful evaluation of symptoms, physical examination, and selected tests. Blood tests and imaging provide valuable information but must be interpreted in the context of the whole clinical picture. Accurate diagnosis allows appropriate treatment and better long-term outcomes.

Action Plan

- Seek evaluation for persistent joint symptoms
- Provide a clear and detailed history
- Do not rely only on lab results
- Follow recommended tests appropriately
- Maintain follow-up if diagnosis is uncertain

A Simple Real-Life Example

A patient came with knee pain and a mildly elevated uric acid level. He believed he had gout.

However, his symptoms were due to osteoarthritis.

Another patient had normal blood tests but clear early rheumatoid arthritis based on symptoms.

Once properly diagnosed, both improved with the correct treatment.

The lesson is simple.

Diagnosis is not just a number. It is the complete story.

Transition to the Next Chapter

Now that you understand how arthritis is diagnosed, the next step is to learn how to manage it in daily life.

In the next chapter, we will discuss the **foundation of arthritis care – lifestyle management**, including weight, daily habits, and practical steps that make a real difference.

CHAPTER 9: Lifestyle Management – The Foundation That Makes Everything Work

Where Real Improvement Begins

When patients hear the word "treatment," they often think first of medicines.

That is understandable. Medicines are visible, quick, and often effective.

But over the years, I have seen a clear pattern.

Patients who depend only on medicines improve partially.
Patients who combine medicines with **daily lifestyle habits** do much better.

Their pain is more controlled. Their movement improves. Their confidence grows.

That is why I tell my patients:

Lifestyle is not an extra step. It is the foundation.

Weight: The Most Practical Place to Start

Let us begin with something simple but powerful.

Body weight.

Every extra pound increases the load on weight-bearing joints, especially the knees and hips.

Patients are often surprised when I explain this.

Even a modest reduction in weight can:

* Reduce joint pain
* Improve mobility
* Decrease stress on joints
* Slow progression of damage

This is not about strict dieting.

It is about **steady, realistic change** that you can maintain.

Joint Protection: Small Changes, Big Impact

Many daily activities place unnecessary strain on joints.

The goal is not to avoid activity.
The goal is to **perform activity wisely**.

Simple principles include:

- Use larger joints instead of smaller ones when possible
- Avoid repetitive strain
- Maintain proper posture
- Distribute weight evenly

For example, lifting an object with both hands instead of one reduces stress on smaller joints.

These small adjustments, repeated daily, make a significant difference.

Activity Pacing: Finding the Right Balance

One of the most common patterns I see is imbalance.

Some patients do too much on good days and suffer afterward. Others avoid activity entirely out of fear.

Both approaches create problems.

A better strategy is pacing.

- Break tasks into smaller parts
- Take short, regular breaks
- Avoid long periods of strain

This allows you to remain active without overloading your joints.

Movement: Essential for Joint Health

Many patients believe that resting a painful joint is the safest option.

Short rest may help during severe pain.

But prolonged inactivity leads to:

- Increased stiffness
- Muscle weakness
- Reduced flexibility

Regular movement:

- Maintains joint flexibility
- Improves circulation
- Strengthens muscles
- Reduces stiffness

The joint is designed to move.

When it stops moving, problems increase.

Sleep: An Underestimated Tool

Sleep is often overlooked in arthritis care.

Poor sleep leads to:

- Increased pain sensitivity

- Reduced energy
- Slower recovery

Good sleep supports healing.

Simple steps include:

- Maintaining a regular sleep schedule
- Using proper pillows and support
- Creating a comfortable sleep environment
- Avoiding stimulants late in the day

Improving sleep often improves pain control.

Stress: The Silent Amplifier

Stress affects how the body experiences pain.

It can:

- Increase muscle tension
- Heighten pain perception
- Trigger flare-ups

Managing stress does not require complicated methods.

Simple techniques help:

- Deep breathing
- Relaxation exercises
- Meditation
- Engaging in enjoyable activities

A calm mind supports a more comfortable body.

Making Your Home Joint-Friendly

Your environment can either support or strain your joints.

Consider simple adjustments:

- Use chairs with good support
- Keep frequently used items within reach
- Use tools that reduce strain on hands
- Ensure safe walking surfaces

These small changes make daily life easier and safer.

Doctor's Pearl

Consistency matters more than intensity.

You do not need dramatic changes.
Small, steady improvements practiced daily bring the best results.

Myth vs Fact

Myth: Lifestyle changes do not make much difference.
Fact: Lifestyle is one of the most powerful tools in arthritis care.

Myth: Resting protects joints.
Fact: Controlled movement is essential.

Common Mistakes to Avoid

- Ignoring weight management
- Avoiding activity completely
- Overexerting on good days
- Neglecting sleep
- Ignoring stress

Red Flag Warnings

Seek guidance if you notice:

- Rapid decline in mobility
- Severe pain with minimal activity
- Difficulty performing daily tasks
- Persistent sleep problems
- Increasing dependence

Key Points

- Lifestyle is the foundation of arthritis care

- Weight control reduces joint stress
- Joint protection prevents damage
- Balanced activity maintains function
- Sleep and stress management are essential

Chapter Summary

Lifestyle plays a central role in managing arthritis. Weight control, joint protection, balanced activity, proper sleep, and stress management significantly improve symptoms and quality of life. These measures enhance the effect of medical treatment and support long-term joint health.

Action Plan

- Aim for gradual weight control
- Practice joint protection daily
- Stay active with balanced movement
- Improve sleep habits
- Manage stress regularly
- Make small home adjustments

A Simple Real-Life Example

A patient with knee arthritis relied mainly on medicines but continued to struggle.

We focused on simple lifestyle changes. Modest weight loss, regular walking, and better pacing.

Over time, his pain reduced, and his function improved.

He told me, "Doctor, I did not realize simple habits could help this much."

That is the power of consistency.

Transition to the Next Chapter

Now that you understand the importance of lifestyle, the next step is to focus on one of the most effective tools available.

In the next chapter, we will explore **exercise and physical therapy**, and how movement can be used as medicine.

CHAPTER 10: Exercise and Physical Therapy – Using Movement as Medicine

The Fear That Holds Many People Back

When I advise patients with arthritis to exercise, I often see hesitation.

"Doctor, won't exercise damage my joints?"

It is a very natural concern.

But the truth is reassuring and important:

The right kind of movement protects your joints. Avoiding movement often harms them.

Over the years, I have seen patients improve significantly, not because of stronger medicines, but because they learned how to move correctly and consistently.

Exercise is not just an option.
It is a **core part of treatment**.

What Happens When You Stop Moving

Let us first understand what inactivity does.

When movement decreases:

- Muscles become weak
- Joints become stiff
- Balance worsens
- Pain often increases

A cycle begins:

Less movement leads to stiffness
Stiffness increases discomfort
Discomfort leads to even less movement

Breaking this cycle is one of the most important steps in managing arthritis.

The Three Types of Exercise You Need

A balanced exercise plan includes three types of movement. Each plays a different role.

---

1. Range-of-Motion Exercises

These are gentle movements that keep joints flexible.

They help to:

- Reduce stiffness
- Maintain joint mobility
- Prevent tightness

Examples include:

- Gentle stretching
- Slow bending and straightening of joints

These exercises can usually be done daily.

2. Strengthening Exercises

These exercises build muscle strength around the joint.

Strong muscles:

- Support the joint
- Reduce stress on cartilage
- Improve stability

Examples include:

- Light resistance band exercises
- Sit-to-stand movements
- Simple leg or arm strengthening

You do not need heavy weights. Consistency matters more than intensity.

3. Aerobic (Endurance) Exercise

These activities improve overall fitness.

They help to:

- Improve heart health
- Support weight control
- Increase energy

Examples include:

- Walking
- Cycling
- Swimming

A combination of all three types gives the best results.

How to Start Safely

One of the most common mistakes is doing too much too quickly.

A better approach is simple:

- Start slowly
- Increase gradually
- Stay consistent
- Listen to your body

Mild discomfort may occur in the beginning.

But sharp or worsening pain is a signal to stop and adjust.

CHAPTER 10
MOVEMENT IS MEDICINE

1. FLEXIBILITY

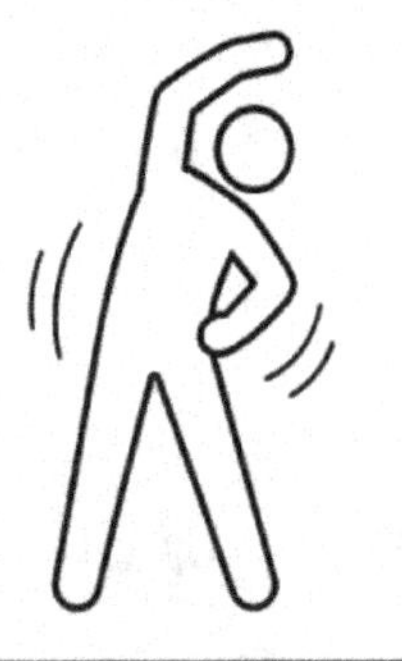

- STRETCH DAILY
- REDUCE STIFFNESS

2. STRENGTH

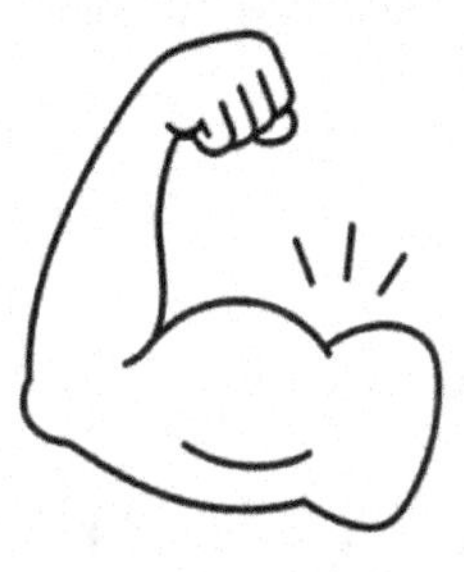

- STRONG MUSCLES SUPPORT JOINTS

3. ENDURANCE

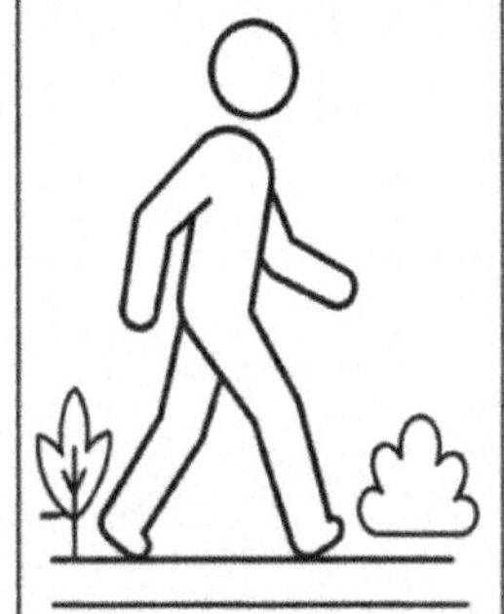

- WALK OR CYCLE REGULARLY

MOVE DAILY

MOVE GENTLY

MOVE CONSISTENTLY

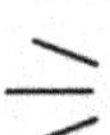 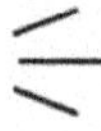 Movement reduces pain and improves mobility.

The Role of Physical Therapy

For many patients, especially in the beginning, physical therapy is very helpful.

A trained therapist can:

- Design a personalized exercise plan
- Teach correct technique
- Improve posture and movement patterns
- Prevent injury

This guidance builds confidence and ensures safety.

Low-Impact Activities: Gentle but Effective

Not all exercise is suitable for every joint.

Low-impact activities are often the best choice.

These include:

- Walking
- Swimming
- Water-based exercises
- Cycling
- Gentle yoga

Water exercises are especially helpful because they reduce stress on joints while allowing movement.

Exercising During Flare-Ups

Patients often ask, "Should I stop exercising during a flare?"

The answer depends on severity.

- During mild flare-ups: gentle movement can help
- During severe flare-ups: reduce intensity and rest more

Complete inactivity should be avoided if possible.

The key is to **adjust, not stop completely**.

Common Exercise Mistakes

I often see these patterns:

- Doing too much on the first day
- Avoiding exercise out of fear
- Using incorrect technique
- Ignoring warning signs
- Being inconsistent

Consistency is far more important than intensity.

Doctor's Pearl

Movement is medicine.

When used correctly, it reduces pain, improves function, and protects your joints.

Myth vs Fact

Myth: Exercise damages arthritic joints.
Fact: Proper exercise strengthens and protects joints.

Myth: Rest is better than movement.
Fact: Controlled movement is essential.

Common Mistakes to Avoid

- Remaining inactive due to fear
- Starting with high-intensity exercise
- Ignoring guidance
- Stopping exercise too early
- Skipping warm-up and cool-down

Red Flag Warnings

Stop and seek advice if you notice:

- Sudden severe pain
- Increasing swelling after exercise
- Joint instability

- Dizziness or imbalance
- Pain that does not improve with rest

Key Points

- Exercise is a key part of treatment
- Flexibility, strength, and endurance all matter
- Start slowly and progress gradually
- Physical therapy can guide safe exercise
- Consistency is essential

Chapter Summary

Exercise plays a central role in managing arthritis. It improves flexibility, strengthens muscles, enhances overall fitness, and reduces pain. A balanced approach that includes range-of-motion, strengthening, and aerobic exercises provides the best results. Starting slowly and maintaining consistency are the keys to long-term success.

Action Plan

- Begin with gentle daily movement
- Add simple stretching exercises
- Include light strengthening exercises
- Walk regularly or choose another low-impact activity

- Consider physical therapy if needed
- Stay consistent

A Simple Real-Life Example

A patient with knee arthritis avoided exercise because he feared worsening his pain.

Over time, his muscles weakened, and his symptoms increased.

We started with short walks and basic strengthening exercises.

Within weeks, his strength improved, and his pain reduced.

He told me, "Doctor, I should have started earlier."

Transition to the Next Chapter

Now that you understand how movement can help your joints, the next step is to look at another powerful factor.

In the next chapter, we will discuss **food, weight, and inflammation**, and how your daily diet can support your joint health.

CHAPTER 11: Food, Weight, and Inflammation – Eating in a Way That Helps Your Joints

A Question Almost Every Patient Asks

Sooner or later, almost every patient asks me:

"Doctor, what should I eat for my arthritis?"

It is a very natural question. Food is something we choose every day. It feels logical that the right diet should help.

Let me give you a clear and honest answer.

Diet alone does not cure most types of arthritis. But the right eating habits can make a **real and meaningful difference**.

They can reduce inflammation, help control weight, improve energy, and support overall health.

Think of diet not as a cure, but as a **powerful partner** in your treatment.

The Weight–Joint Connection

Before discussing specific foods, we must understand something very important.

Your body weight has a direct effect on your joints.

Every extra pound increases the load on weight-bearing joints such as the knees and hips.

Over time, this leads to:

- Increased joint stress
- Faster cartilage wear
- More pain
- Reduced mobility

Even modest weight reduction can:

- Reduce pain
- Improve function
- Slow disease progression

This is one of the most practical and effective ways to help your joints.

What Does "Anti-Inflammatory Eating" Mean?

You may have heard the term "anti-inflammatory diet."

It may sound complicated, but it is actually quite simple.

It means choosing foods that:

- Support natural body balance
- Reduce unnecessary inflammation
- Provide steady energy

This is not about strict rules.

It is about **consistent, sensible choices** over time.

Foods That Support Joint Health

Certain foods are generally helpful for overall health and may support joint function.

These include:

- Fruits and vegetables rich in antioxidants
- Whole grains for steady energy
- Healthy fats such as those from nuts, seeds, and olive oil
- Fish rich in omega-3 fatty acids
- Legumes such as beans and lentils

No single food is a solution. But together, these choices create a healthier internal environment.

Foods That May Worsen Symptoms

Some foods may increase inflammation or worsen symptoms in certain individuals.

These include:

- Highly processed foods
- Excess sugar
- Refined carbohydrates
- Processed and red meats in excess
- Sugary beverages

You do not need to eliminate everything completely.

The goal is moderation and balance, not strict restriction.

Special Considerations in Gout

In gout, diet plays a more direct role.

Certain foods can increase uric acid levels and trigger attacks.

Helpful measures include:

- Limiting red meat and organ meats
- Reducing alcohol, especially beer
- Avoiding high-fructose drinks
- Drinking adequate water

Even here, diet is only one part of treatment, but it is an important part.

What About Supplements?

Many patients ask about supplements.

Common ones include:

- Omega-3 fatty acids
- Vitamin D
- Calcium
- Glucosamine and chondroitin

Some patients feel benefit, others do not.

The important point is this:

Supplements are **not a substitute for proper treatment**.
They should be used thoughtfully and preferably with medical advice.

Hydration: A Simple but Important Habit

Adequate fluid intake is often overlooked.

Good hydration:

- Supports overall body function
- Helps joint health
- Assists in conditions like gout

This is one of the simplest habits with meaningful benefits.

CHAPTER 11
FOOD & JOINT HEALTH

1. HEALTHY FOOD

- Vegetables
- Protein
- Whole grains

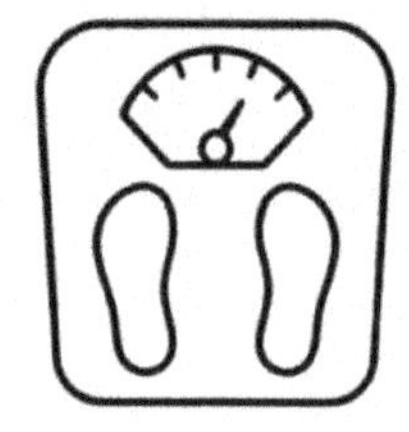

2. WEIGHT CONTROL

- Less weight
- Less joint stress

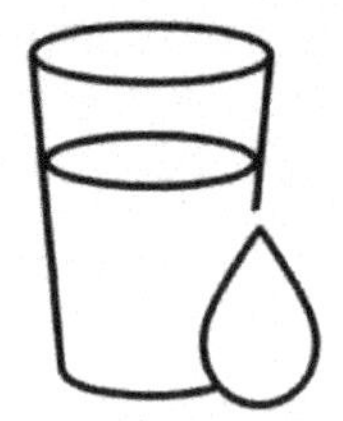

3. HYDRATION

- Drink enough water

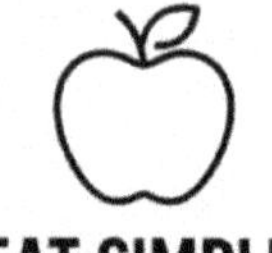

EAT SIMPLE

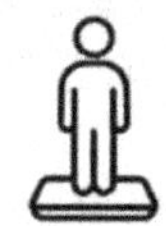

STAY LIGHT

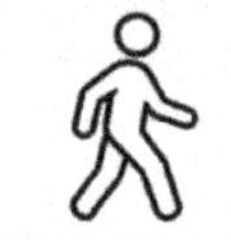

STAY ACTIVE

 **Healthy weight reduces joint pain** 

Keep It Practical and Sustainable

Many patients feel overwhelmed when trying to follow a "perfect diet."

Perfection is not necessary.

What works better is a **practical and sustainable approach**:

- Choose fresh foods when possible
- Include vegetables in most meals
- Maintain balanced portions
- Avoid extreme diets
- Be consistent

Small, steady changes are more effective than short-term strict plans.

Doctor's Pearl

Do not chase miracle diets.

A simple, balanced eating pattern followed consistently is far more effective.

Myth vs Fact

Myth: There is a special diet that can cure arthritis.
Fact: Diet supports management but does not cure most forms.

Myth: Supplements can replace medications.
Fact: Supplements may help but cannot replace proper treatment.

Common Mistakes to Avoid

- Following extreme diets
- Ignoring weight management
- Overusing supplements
- Eating excessive processed foods
- Being inconsistent

Red Flag Warnings

Seek medical advice if:

- You plan major dietary changes
- You have frequent gout attacks
- You have significant weight changes
- You have other conditions such as diabetes or kidney disease

---

Key Points

- Diet plays a supportive role in arthritis care
- Weight control is one of the most important factors
- Balanced eating helps reduce inflammation
- Certain foods may worsen symptoms
- Consistency matters more than perfection

Chapter Summary

Diet and nutrition influence arthritis through their effects on weight, inflammation, and overall health. While diet alone does not cure arthritis, balanced and consistent eating habits can reduce symptoms and improve quality of life. Weight control and hydration are especially important.

Action Plan

- Aim for gradual weight control
- Increase fruits and vegetables
- Include healthy fats and lean proteins
- Reduce processed and sugary foods
- Stay well hydrated
- Follow a sustainable eating pattern

A Simple Real-Life Example

A patient with knee arthritis struggled with persistent pain and excess weight.

Instead of following a strict diet, we focused on simple changes.

He reduced sugary drinks, increased vegetables, and started walking regularly.

Over a few months, he lost some weight and noticed a clear improvement in pain.

He told me, "Doctor, I thought I needed a special diet. Simple changes worked."

Transition to the Next Chapter

Now that you understand how food and weight influence arthritis, the next step is to learn how to manage pain in practical ways.

In the next chapter, we will discuss **how to control arthritis pain without relying heavily on strong medicines**.

CHAPTER 12: Managing Arthritis Pain Without Strong Medicines – Practical Relief That Works

A Concern I Hear Often

Many patients tell me, sometimes with hesitation:

"Doctor, I do not want to depend on strong medicines."

That concern is understandable.

Medicines have a role, and we will use them when needed. But there is something very reassuring you should know.

A large part of arthritis pain can be managed with simple, non-drug methods.

In fact, when used consistently, these methods often reduce the need for stronger medications.

This chapter is about giving you **practical tools you can use every day**.

Heat and Cold: Simple, Effective, and Underused

One of the easiest ways to reduce pain is by using
temperature.

Heat Therapy

Heat helps by:

- Relaxing muscles
- Reducing stiffness
- Improving blood flow

It is especially useful for:

- Morning stiffness
- Chronic tightness
- Muscle discomfort around joints

Simple methods include:

- Warm showers
- Heating pads
- Warm compresses

Cold Therapy

Cold works differently.

It helps by:

- Reducing inflammation
- Numbing the painful area
- Controlling swelling

It is useful for:

- Sudden flare-ups
- Swollen joints
- Recent strain

Cold packs are usually applied for short periods, about 10 to 15 minutes.

Knowing when to use heat and when to use cold can make a noticeable difference.

Topical Treatments: Relief Where You Need It

Topical treatments are applied directly over the painful joint.

These include:

- Pain-relieving gels
- Anti-inflammatory creams
- Capsaicin-based products

They provide local relief with fewer whole-body side effects compared to tablets.

They are especially helpful for joints like the knees and hands.

CHAPTER 12

PAIN RELIEF

WITHOUT STRONG MEDICINES

1.
HEAT

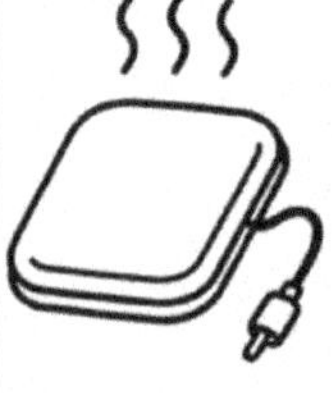

Relieves
stiffness

2.
COLD

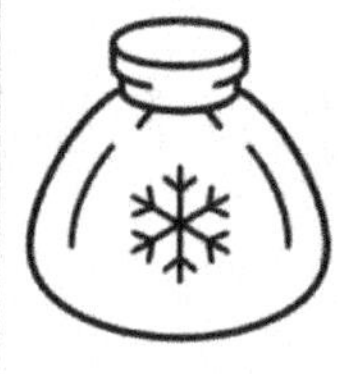

Reduces
swelling

3.
SUPPORT

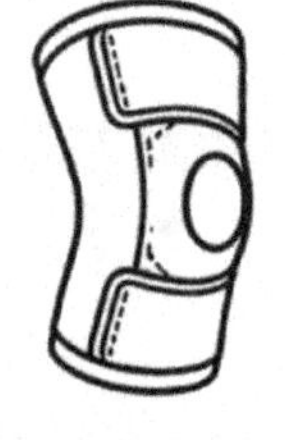

Protect
joints

4.
**REST &
RELAX**

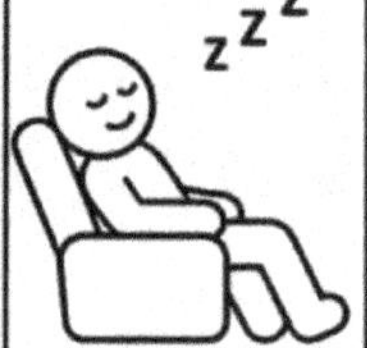

Reduce
pain

 **USE SIMPLE METHODS FIRST** 

Less medicines, safer relief

Braces and Supports: Reducing Stress on Joints

Sometimes, a joint simply needs support.

Using braces or supports can:

- Reduce strain
- Improve alignment
- Increase stability
- Make movement more comfortable

Examples include:

- Knee braces
- Wrist supports
- Shoe inserts
- A walking cane when needed

These aids often improve confidence and mobility.

Activity Modification: Doing Things the Smart Way

Pain is often influenced by how we use our joints.

Simple changes can reduce stress:

- Avoid prolonged standing or sitting
- Take regular breaks
- Break large tasks into smaller steps

- Use proper body mechanics

You do not need to stop your activities.

You need to **do them in a joint-friendly way**.

Mind-Body Techniques: Calming the Pain Response

Pain is not only physical. The mind plays an important role.

Stress and anxiety can increase pain perception.

Helpful techniques include:

- Deep breathing
- Relaxation exercises
- Meditation
- Gentle mindfulness practices

These methods:

- Reduce pain sensitivity
- Improve coping
- Promote calmness

They are simple, safe, and effective when practiced regularly.

Sleep: Breaking the Pain Cycle

Poor sleep increases pain. Pain disrupts sleep.

This creates a difficult cycle.

Improving sleep helps:

- Reduce pain sensitivity
- Improve energy
- Enhance recovery

Helpful steps include:

- Keeping a regular sleep schedule
- Using comfortable support
- Avoiding late-night stimulants
- Creating a calm sleep environment

Better sleep often leads to better pain control.

Gentle Therapies: Additional Support

Many patients benefit from:

- Gentle massage
- Warm water therapy
- Stretching

These methods help:

- Relax muscles
- Improve circulation
- Reduce stiffness

They work best when combined with other strategies.

Doctor's Pearl

Pain control is not about one single method.

It is about combining small, effective steps and using them consistently.

Myth vs Fact

Myth: Strong medicines are the only way to control arthritis pain.
Fact: Many non-drug methods can significantly reduce pain.

Myth: Nothing helps unless the pain is completely gone.
Fact: Even partial relief can greatly improve daily life.

Common Mistakes to Avoid

- Relying only on medicines
- Using heat or cold incorrectly
- Ignoring supportive devices

- Neglecting sleep and stress
- Expecting instant results

Red Flag Warnings

Seek medical advice if you notice:

- Sudden severe pain
- Increasing swelling
- Pain that does not improve
- Joint instability
- Difficulty performing daily activities

Key Points

- Non-drug methods are effective
- Heat helps stiffness, cold helps swelling
- Topical treatments provide local relief
- Supports reduce joint stress
- Sleep and stress management are important

Chapter Summary

Arthritis pain can often be managed effectively without strong medicines. Heat and cold therapy, topical treatments, supportive devices, activity modification, and mind-body techniques all play important roles. When used together and consistently, these methods improve comfort and reduce reliance on medications.

Action Plan

- Use heat for stiffness and cold for swelling
- Try topical treatments for local pain
- Use braces or supports when needed
- Practice relaxation techniques
- Improve sleep habits
- Modify daily activities

A Simple Real-Life Example

A patient with hand arthritis relied heavily on pain medicines but continued to struggle.

We introduced simple measures. Warm water soaks, topical gel, and better joint protection.

Within weeks, her pain reduced, and she needed fewer medicines.

She told me, "Doctor, these simple steps helped more than I expected."

Transition to the Next Chapter

Now that you understand how to manage pain without strong medicines, the next step is to understand how medicines can be used safely when needed.

In the next chapter, we will discuss **basic medicines used in arthritis and how to use them wisely**.

CHAPTER 13: Medicines for Arthritis – Using Them Wisely, Safely, and Effectively

Finding the Right Balance

By now, you understand that lifestyle, movement, and daily habits form the foundation of arthritis care.

But there are times when these are not enough.

Pain may persist. Inflammation may continue. Daily activities may become difficult.

This is where medicines play an important role.

Let me say this clearly.

Medicines are not something to fear. They are something to use wisely.

When used properly, they reduce pain, control inflammation, and help you stay active. When misused, they can lead to avoidable problems.

The goal is not to avoid medicines.
The goal is to use them **correctly and thoughtfully**.

What Are We Trying to Achieve?

Before choosing any medicine, we must be clear about the goal.

Medicines are used to:

- Reduce pain
- Decrease inflammation
- Improve movement
- Prevent long-term joint damage in certain conditions

Not all medicines do all of these things.

That is why treatment must be individualized.

Acetaminophen: A Simple Starting Point

For mild to moderate pain, acetaminophen is often used.

It:

- Reduces pain
- Has minimal effect on inflammation
- Is generally safe when used within recommended limits

It is commonly used in osteoarthritis.

However, higher-than-recommended doses can affect the liver. So it must always be used carefully.

Topical NSAIDs: Local Treatment with Less Risk

Topical nonsteroidal anti-inflammatory drugs are applied directly to the skin over the joint.

They:

- Reduce pain and inflammation locally
- Have fewer systemic side effects than tablets
- Are especially useful for knees and hands

For many patients, this is a practical and safer option.

Oral NSAIDs: Effective but Require Caution

Oral NSAIDs, such as ibuprofen and naproxen, are widely used.

They:

- Reduce pain
- Decrease inflammation
- Improve function

However, they must be used carefully.

Possible risks include effects on:

- The stomach (ulcers, bleeding)
- The kidneys
- The heart in some individuals

They should be used:

- At the lowest effective dose
- For the shortest necessary duration
- Under medical guidance, especially in older adults

Steroids: Powerful but Not for Long-Term Use

Steroids are strong anti-inflammatory medicines.

They may be given:

- Orally
- As injections into joints

They are very effective for short-term control.

However, long-term use may lead to:

- Weight gain
- Increased blood sugar
- Bone loss
- Increased risk of infection

They are useful, but should be used **carefully and for appropriate durations**.

MEDICINES FOR ARTHRITIS

Use the Right Medicine, the Right Way

1 PAIN RELIEVERS

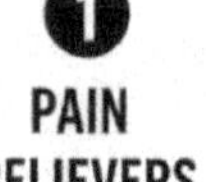

- Reduce pain and inflammation
- Use only as needed

2 ANTI-INFLAMMATORY MEDICINES

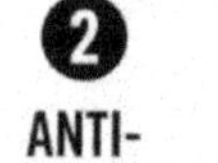

- Reduce swelling and pain
- Take with food as advised

3 DMARDs (DISEASE MODIFYING)

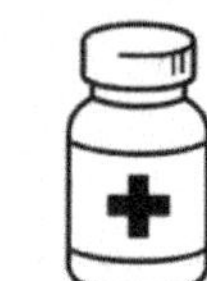

- Slow down disease progression
- Take regularly as prescribed

4 TOPICAL MEDICINES

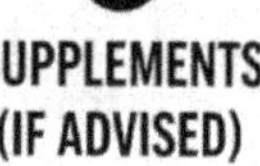

- Creams, gels or patches
- Helpful for local pain

5 SUPPLEMENTS (IF ADVISED)

- Calcium, Vitamin D and others
- Support bone and joint health

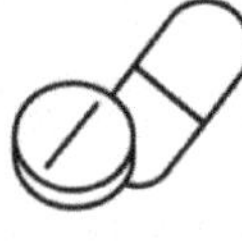
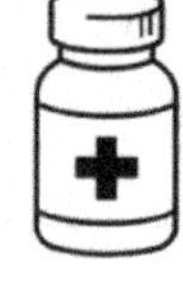
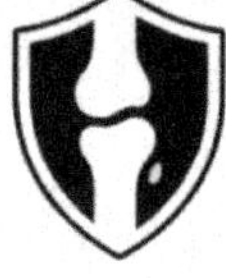
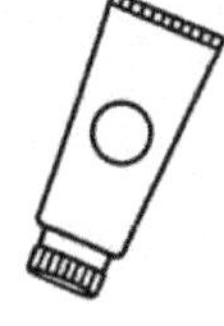
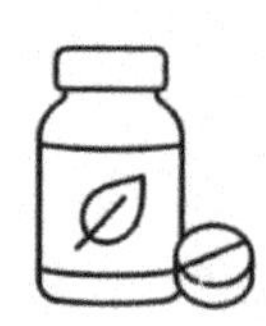

IMPORTANT REMINDERS

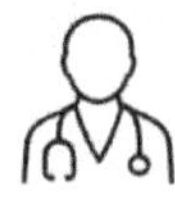

Follow your doctor's advice

Take medicines at the right time

Do not stop medicine suddenly

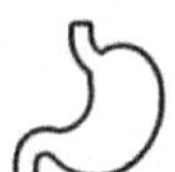

Watch for side effects and report early

Regular check-up for safe and effective use

MEDICINES WORK BEST WITH

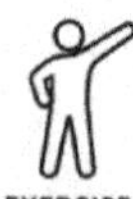

EXERCISE

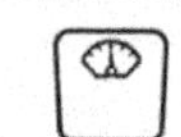

WEIGHT CONTROL

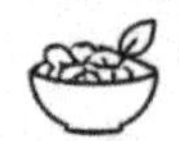

HEALTHY DIET

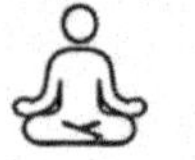

STRESS MANAGEMENT

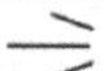 **RIGHT MEDICINE + RIGHT USE = BETTER RELIEF, BETTER LIFE** 

Joint Injections: Targeted Relief

Injecting medication directly into the joint can provide relief in selected cases.

These are often used for:

- Knee arthritis
- Shoulder problems
- Local flare-ups

They can reduce inflammation and improve function.

The effect is usually temporary, but often very helpful.

Safety in Older Adults

Many patients with arthritis are older.

This makes careful use of medicines even more important.

Factors to consider include:

- Kidney function
- Risk of stomach problems
- Interaction with other medications

Even commonly used medicines are not completely harmless.

They must be used with awareness.

Principles of Safe Use

A few simple rules help ensure safe treatment:

- Use the lowest effective dose
- Avoid combining similar medicines without advice
- Do not use medicines for long periods without review
- Inform your doctor about all medications you take
- Watch for side effects

Medicines should support your overall plan, not replace it.

Doctor's Pearl

The best treatment is not the strongest medicine.

It is the **right medicine, used in the right way, at the right time**.

Myth vs Fact

Myth: If a medicine works, taking more will help more.
Fact: Higher doses increase risk without adding benefit.

Myth: Over-the-counter medicines are completely safe.
Fact: They can cause serious side effects if misused.

Common Mistakes to Avoid

- Self-medicating for long periods
- Taking multiple pain medicines together
- Ignoring side effects
- Using higher doses than needed
- Not informing your doctor about all medications

Red Flag Warnings

Seek medical advice if you notice:

- Stomach pain or bleeding
- Swelling of legs
- Reduced urine output
- Unusual fatigue
- New symptoms after starting a medicine

Key Points

- Medicines play an important role in arthritis care
- Different medicines have different purposes
- NSAIDs are effective but require caution
- Steroids are powerful but should be limited
- Safe use and monitoring are essential

Chapter Summary

Medicines help manage arthritis by reducing pain and inflammation. Options include acetaminophen, topical and oral NSAIDs, steroids, and joint injections. Each has benefits and risks. Proper use requires careful selection, appropriate dosing, and monitoring. Medicines work best when combined with lifestyle and non-drug measures.

Action Plan

- Use medicines as prescribed
- Prefer topical options when suitable
- Avoid long-term unsupervised use
- Monitor for side effects
- Combine medicines with lifestyle measures
- Maintain regular follow-up

A Simple Real-Life Example

A patient was taking multiple pain medicines daily without proper guidance.

Over time, he developed stomach discomfort and early kidney problems.

We simplified his treatment, reduced unnecessary medicines, and added safer options.

His pain remained controlled, but his overall risk decreased.

The lesson is simple.

Wise use of medicines protects both your joints and your overall health.

Transition to the Next Chapter

Now that you understand the basic medicines used in arthritis, the next step is to learn about treatments that go deeper.

In the next chapter, we will discuss **advanced therapies that can control the disease and prevent long-term damage**.

CHAPTER 14: Advanced Treatments – Controlling the Disease at Its Root

When Basic Treatment Is Not Enough

Up to this point, we have focused on reducing pain, improving movement, and supporting daily function.

For many patients, especially those with osteoarthritis, these steps are sufficient for a long time.

But in some types of arthritis, particularly **inflammatory arthritis**, the problem goes deeper.

It is not just pain.

It is **ongoing inflammation that can silently damage the joints**.

In these situations, simply controlling symptoms is not enough.

We must control the **disease process itself**.

Understanding "Disease-Modifying" Treatment

You may hear the term DMARDs, which stands for Disease-Modifying Anti-Rheumatic Drugs.

This may sound complex, but the idea is simple.

These medicines:

- Target the underlying disease
- Reduce inflammation at a deeper level
- Slow or prevent joint damage

This is different from pain medicines, which mainly provide symptom relief.

This difference is very important.

Methotrexate: A Key Treatment

Methotrexate is one of the most commonly used medicines in inflammatory arthritis, especially rheumatoid arthritis.

It:

- Reduces inflammation
- Controls disease activity
- Helps prevent joint damage

It is usually taken once a week and requires regular monitoring.

When used appropriately, many patients do very well with this medicine.

Other Conventional DMARDs

Depending on the condition, other medicines may be used along with or instead of methotrexate.

These include:

- Sulfasalazine
- Hydroxychloroquine
- Leflunomide

Treatment is tailored based on:

- Disease severity
- Patient characteristics
- Response to therapy

There is no one-size-fits-all approach.

Biologic Therapies: Targeted Treatment

Biologic medicines are a major advancement in arthritis care.

They are designed to target specific parts of the immune system.

These treatments:

- Are used when conventional DMARDs are not sufficient
- Are given as injections or infusions
- Can provide significant improvement

For many patients, biologics have changed the course of disease and improved quality of life.

JAK Inhibitors: A Newer Option

JAK inhibitors are a newer class of medications.

They:

- Target specific pathways involved in inflammation
- Are taken as tablets
- Offer an alternative when other treatments are not suitable

They represent another step forward in treatment options.

Gout: Treating the Root Cause

In gout, long-term treatment focuses on reducing uric acid levels.

Medicines such as:

- Allopurinol

- Febuxostat

help prevent repeated attacks and joint damage.

Managing gout is not only about treating pain.
It is about controlling the underlying cause.

Monitoring and Safety

Advanced treatments require careful monitoring.

This may include:

- Regular blood tests
- Checking liver and kidney function
- Monitoring blood counts
- Watching for signs of infection

This does not mean these medicines are unsafe.

It means they must be used **responsibly and under supervision**.

When to See a Specialist

In many cases, especially inflammatory arthritis,
specialist care is important.

You should consider seeing a rheumatologist if:

- Symptoms suggest inflammatory arthritis
- Diagnosis is unclear
- Symptoms are not well controlled
- Advanced treatment is needed

Early specialist care often leads to better long-term outcomes.

Doctor's Pearl

In inflammatory arthritis, timing is critical.

Starting the right treatment early can prevent permanent joint damage.

Delaying treatment may allow damage that cannot be reversed.

Myth vs Fact

Myth: Strong medicines should be avoided as long as possible.
Fact: Early use of appropriate treatment can prevent serious damage.

Myth: If pain improves, the disease is controlled.
Fact: Disease activity may continue even when pain decreases.

Common Mistakes to Avoid

- Delaying advanced treatment
- Stopping medicines without advice
- Ignoring monitoring requirements
- Focusing only on pain relief
- Avoiding specialist consultation

Red Flag Warnings

Seek medical advice if you notice:

- Persistent joint swelling despite treatment
- Worsening symptoms
- Side effects from medicines
- Signs of infection
- Unexplained fatigue

Key Points

- Advanced treatments target the disease itself
- DMARDs help prevent joint damage
- Biologic therapies provide targeted control
- Gout requires long-term uric acid management
- Monitoring is essential

Chapter Summary

Advanced treatments are essential for certain types of arthritis, especially inflammatory conditions. These therapies aim to control the disease process and prevent long-term damage. Proper use, monitoring, and timely initiation are key to achieving the best outcomes.

Action Plan

- Understand the purpose of advanced treatments
- Do not delay recommended therapy
- Follow monitoring schedules
- Report side effects promptly
- Seek specialist care when needed
- Stay consistent with treatment

A Simple Real-Life Example

A patient with early rheumatoid arthritis hesitated to start methotrexate due to fear of strong medicines.

After discussion, he agreed to begin treatment.

Within months, his symptoms improved, and over time, joint damage was prevented.

Another patient delayed treatment and later developed joint deformities.

The difference was not the disease.

The difference was **timely action**.

Transition to the Next Chapter

Now that you understand advanced treatments, the next step is to explore situations where medicines may not be enough.

In the next chapter, we will discuss **surgical options**, including when they are needed and what to expect.

CHAPTER 15: Surgical Treatment – When It Becomes the Right Choice

Facing the Idea of Surgery

At some point, many patients ask me, often with hesitation:

"Doctor, will I need surgery?"

It is a question that carries concern, sometimes even fear.

Let me begin with reassurance.

Most patients with arthritis do not need surgery.

With proper care, many people manage well for years with lifestyle changes, exercise, and medications.

However, there are situations where surgery becomes not just helpful, but **transformative**.

The key is understanding **when it is truly needed**.

When Should Surgery Be Considered?

Surgery is not the first step. It is considered when other treatments no longer provide enough relief.

You may consider surgery if:

- Pain is severe and persistent
- Daily activities become difficult
- Movement is significantly limited
- Medicines and other treatments are no longer effective
- Quality of life is clearly affected

The decision is not based on X-rays alone.

It is based on how much your life is being affected.

Joint Replacement: The Most Common and Effective Option

Joint replacement is one of the most successful procedures in modern medicine.

In this procedure:

- The damaged parts of the joint are removed
- Artificial components replace them

It is most commonly done for:

- Knees
- Hips

It may also be done for shoulders and other joints in selected cases.

Benefits

- Significant pain relief
- Improved movement
- Better quality of life

Many patients return to normal or near-normal activities after recovery.

Arthroscopy: Limited but Useful in Selected Cases

Arthroscopy uses a small camera to examine and treat problems inside a joint.

It may be helpful in specific situations such as:

- Certain cartilage injuries
- Meniscal problems

However, in advanced osteoarthritis, its benefit is limited.

Avoiding unnecessary procedures is important.

SURGICAL TREATMENTS FOR ARTHRITIS

When Surgery May Help

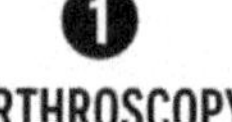

① ARTHROSCOPY

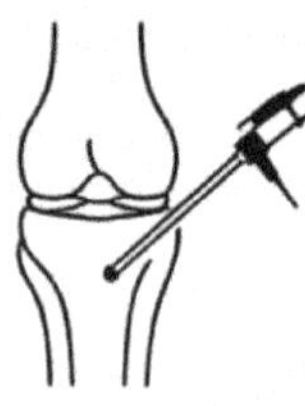

- Keyhole surgery to clean or repair the joint
- Less pain, faster recovery

② OSTEOTOMY

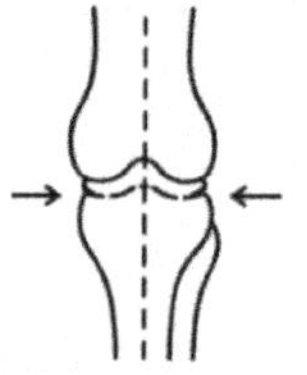

- Realigns bone to reduce pain
- Delays need for joint replacement

③ PARTIAL JOINT REPLACEMENT

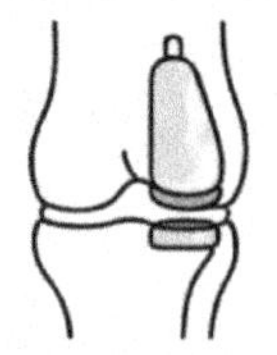

- Replaces only the damaged part
- More natural movement

④ TOTAL JOINT REPLACEMENT

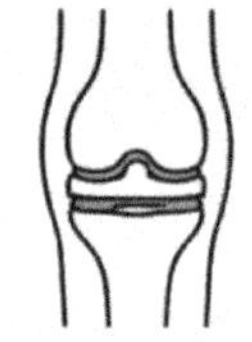

- Replaces the entire joint
- Best option for severe arthritis

BENEFITS OF SURGERY

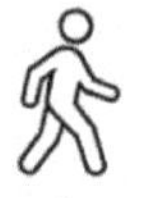

REDUCES PAIN

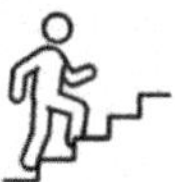

IMPROVES MOVEMENT

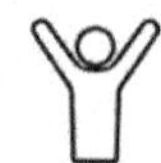

BETTER QUALITY OF LIFE

LONG-LASTING RELIEF

IMPORTANT TO REMEMBER

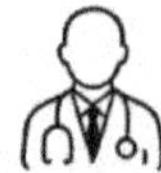

CONSULT YOUR ORTHOPEDIC SPECIALIST

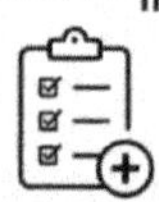

EVALUATE YOUR CONDITION CAREFULLY

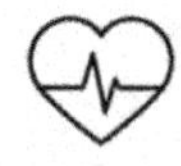

FOLLOW DOCTOR'S ADVICE BEFORE SURGERY

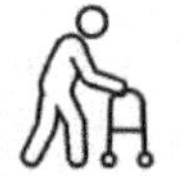

REHABILITATION IS KEY TO RECOVERY

SURGERY IS SAFE AND EFFECTIVE

THE RIGHT SURGERY CAN GIVE YOU A PAIN-FREE, ACTIVE LIFE

Joint Fusion: Stability Over Movement

In some joints, especially smaller ones, fusion may be considered.

In this procedure:

- Two bones are permanently joined
- Movement is reduced or eliminated
- Pain is decreased

This is usually reserved for specific situations when other options are not suitable.

Other Corrective Procedures

In selected cases, surgery may be done to:

- Realign the joint
- Remove damaged tissue
- Improve joint function

These procedures are less common and depend on individual needs.

What to Expect from Joint Replacement

Understanding the process reduces anxiety.

Before Surgery

- Medical evaluation
- Discussion of risks and benefits
- Planning and preparation

After Surgery

- Gradual pain improvement
- Early start of physical therapy
- Progressive return of movement

Long-Term Outcome

- Significant improvement in most patients
- Artificial joints often last many years

The goal is not perfection.

The goal is **less pain and better function**.

Risks to Keep in Mind

All surgeries carry some risks.

These include:

- Infection
- Blood clots
- Implant-related issues
- Need for repeat surgery in the future

With modern care and proper preparation, these risks are generally low.

Recovery Depends on Your Participation

Surgery is only one part of the process.

Recovery depends on:

- Physical therapy
- Patient effort
- Regular follow-up

Patients who actively participate in rehabilitation usually recover better.

Doctor's Pearl

Surgery is not a failure.

It is a continuation of treatment when other methods are no longer enough.

When done at the right time, it can restore independence.

Myth vs Fact

Myth: Surgery should always be avoided.
Fact: In selected cases, it is the best option.

Myth: Surgery gives instant results.
Fact: Recovery takes time and effort.

Common Mistakes to Avoid

- Delaying surgery despite severe limitation
- Expecting immediate results
- Ignoring rehabilitation
- Making decisions based only on imaging
- Not discussing risks clearly

Red Flag Warnings

Seek medical advice if:

- Pain severely limits daily life
- You cannot walk or perform basic tasks
- Symptoms continue to worsen
- Other treatments no longer help
- Quality of life is significantly reduced

Key Points

- Most patients do not need surgery
- Surgery is considered when other treatments fail

- Joint replacement is the most common procedure
- Rehabilitation is essential for recovery
- Proper timing improves outcomes

Chapter Summary

Surgical treatment is an important option for patients with advanced arthritis who do not respond to other therapies. Joint replacement can provide significant pain relief and improved function. Careful selection, proper timing, and active participation in rehabilitation are key to success.

Action Plan

- Consider surgery only when necessary
- Discuss options thoroughly with your doctor
- Prepare well before surgery
- Follow rehabilitation plans carefully
- Maintain regular follow-up

A Simple Real-Life Example

A patient with severe knee arthritis avoided surgery for years due to fear.

Over time, his mobility declined, and his pain increased.

Eventually, he agreed to knee replacement.

After recovery, he was able to walk comfortably and return to daily activities.

He told me, "Doctor, I waited too long."

Transition to the Next Chapter

Now that you understand when surgery becomes necessary, the next step is to look ahead.

In the next chapter, we will discuss **new and emerging treatments**, and how to separate real progress from unproven claims.

CHAPTER 16: New and Emerging Treatments – Hope, Progress, and the Need for Caution

The Question Behind Every Hope

At some point, almost every patient asks me:

"Doctor, is there anything new that can cure arthritis?"

I understand that question very well.

Living with a long-term condition naturally makes us look for something better. Something that can reverse the problem completely.

The encouraging news is this.

Research in arthritis is active and progressing.

New treatments have already improved the lives of many patients. At the same time, it is important to stay realistic.

**Not everything that is new is proven.
Not everything that is promising is right for you.**

This chapter will help you understand both the possibilities and the limitations.

Regenerative Medicine: Can We Repair the Joint?

One of the most discussed areas today is regenerative medicine.

The idea is simple and appealing.

Instead of only reducing pain, can we **repair damaged joint tissue**?

Two commonly discussed approaches are PRP and stem cell therapy.

Platelet-Rich Plasma (PRP)

PRP is prepared from your own blood and contains growth factors that may support healing.

It is injected into the joint.

Some patients report:

- Reduction in pain
- Improved function, especially in early osteoarthritis

However, results are variable.

Current research shows mixed outcomes, and long-term benefits are still being evaluated.

Stem Cell Therapy

Stem cell therapy aims to regenerate cartilage.

It is an exciting concept, but at present:

- Evidence is still evolving
- Methods are not standardized
- Outcomes are uncertain
- Costs are often high

Some clinics make strong claims that are not always supported by reliable scientific data.

Careful evaluation is essential.

Advances in Biologic Treatments

In inflammatory arthritis, progress has been significant.

Newer biologic therapies:

- Target specific parts of the immune system
- Improve disease control
- Reduce long-term joint damage

For many patients, these treatments have changed the course of disease.

Research continues to refine these therapies further.

JAK Inhibitors and Targeted Therapy

Newer oral medications, such as JAK inhibitors, target specific inflammatory pathways.

They:

- Provide an alternative to injectable treatments
- Offer additional options when other therapies are not sufficient

They represent an important step forward in personalized care.

Personalized Medicine: The Future Direction

Medicine is gradually moving toward a more individualized approach.

In the future, treatment decisions may be guided by:

- Genetic information
- Disease markers
- Individual response patterns

This approach aims to select the most effective treatment for each patient.

While still developing, it holds great promise.

Technology in Arthritis Care

Technology is also becoming part of arthritis management.

You may encounter:

- Mobile applications for symptom tracking
- Wearable devices that monitor activity
- Telemedicine consultations

These tools can help:

- Track progress
- Identify patterns
- Improve communication with healthcare providers

They are helpful additions, though not replacements for medical care.

New Approaches to Pain Control

Researchers are also working on better ways to control pain.

These include:

- Improved topical treatments
- New medications
- Non-drug techniques targeting pain pathways

The goal is to achieve better relief with fewer side effects.

What You Should Be Careful About

With so much information available, it is easy to be misled.

Be cautious about:

- Claims of complete cure
- Very expensive treatments with limited evidence
- Clinics that guarantee results
- Testimonials without scientific backing

If something sounds too good to be true, it usually needs careful evaluation.

Doctor's Pearl

Hope is important.

But it should always be guided by **evidence and careful judgment**.

Myth vs Fact

Myth: New treatments are always better.
Fact: New treatments must be proven safe and effective.

Myth: Regenerative therapies can cure arthritis.
Fact: Most are still under study and are not guaranteed solutions.

Common Mistakes to Avoid

- Chasing unproven treatments
- Ignoring established therapies
- Spending large amounts on uncertain options
- Relying on anecdotal success stories
- Not discussing options with your doctor

Red Flag Warnings

Be cautious if you encounter:

- Guaranteed cure claims
- Lack of clear scientific explanation
- Pressure to make quick decisions
- No discussion of risks
- Very high cost without proven benefit

NEW TREATMENTS FOR ARTHRITIS

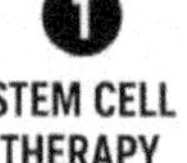
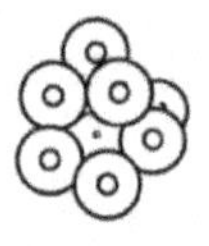

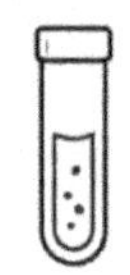
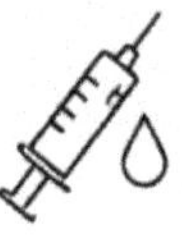

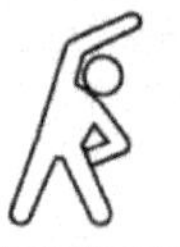

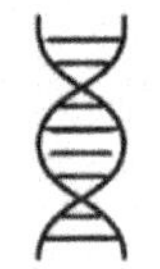

POTENTIAL BENEFITS

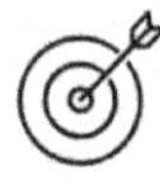
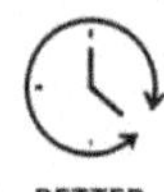
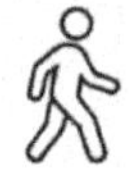

IMPORTANT TO REMEMBER

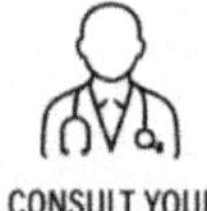

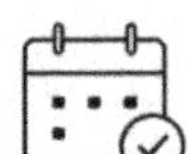

Key Points

- Research in arthritis treatment is advancing
- Regenerative medicine is promising but not fully established
- Biologic therapies have improved outcomes
- Personalized medicine is the future direction
- Careful evaluation is essential

Chapter Summary

New and emerging treatments offer hope for improved arthritis care. Advances in biologic therapies, regenerative medicine, and personalized approaches are shaping the future. However, not all treatments are proven or suitable for every patient. Decisions should always be based on reliable evidence and careful medical guidance.

Action Plan

- Stay informed about new developments
- Discuss options with your doctor
- Evaluate benefits and risks carefully
- Avoid unproven or exaggerated claims
- Focus on evidence-based treatments

A Simple Real-Life Example

A patient once asked about an expensive therapy advertised as a cure for arthritis.

After reviewing the available evidence, he chose to continue with established treatment.

Over time, his symptoms improved, and he avoided unnecessary risk.

He later said, "Doctor, I am glad I did not rush into it."

Transition to the Next Chapter

Now that you understand current and emerging treatments, the next step is to focus on daily life.

In the next chapter, we will discuss **how to live well with arthritis**, manage flare-ups, and maintain independence.

CHAPTER 17: Living Well with Arthritis – Staying Active, Independent, and Positive

Life Does Not Stop Here

When patients first hear the word arthritis, there is often a quiet fear.

"Will I be able to live normally?"
"Will I become dependent on others?"

These are real concerns.

But after many years of caring for patients, I can tell you something important.

Arthritis changes life, but it does not end it.

With the right approach, many people continue to work, travel, care for their families, and enjoy meaningful, fulfilling lives.

The goal is not to remove every symptom.

The goal is to **live well despite the condition.**

Building a Daily Routine That Supports You

A steady routine helps both the body and the mind.

You do not need a complicated plan.

Simple structure works best:

- Begin the day with gentle stretching
- Plan important tasks when your energy is highest
- Take short breaks instead of long periods of strain
- Maintain regular sleep and meal times

Your body responds well to consistency.

Managing Flare-Ups with Confidence

Flare-ups are a natural part of many types of arthritis.

They may feel discouraging, but they do not mean failure.

During a flare:

- Reduce activity temporarily
- Use cold therapy for swelling
- Use heat for stiffness
- Follow your treatment plan
- Rest the joint, but do not completely stop movement

Most flare-ups settle with proper care.

Learning to handle them calmly makes a big difference.

Staying Active Without Overdoing It

Balance is essential.

- Too much activity increases pain
- Too little activity leads to stiffness and weakness

The goal is steady, moderate movement.

Choose:

- Low-impact activities
- Gradual progression
- Regular consistency

Listen to your body. It gives useful feedback.

Maintaining Independence

Independence is deeply important for most people.

Simple adjustments can help preserve it:

- Use supportive chairs and proper footwear
- Keep commonly used items within easy reach
- Use assistive devices when needed
- Modify tasks to reduce strain

These small changes allow you to remain active and
confident.

Emotional Health Matters

Living with a long-term condition affects more than the
body.

You may experience:

- Frustration
- Worry
- Reduced confidence
- Low mood

These feelings are normal.

What matters is how you respond.

Helpful steps include:

- Staying connected with family and friends
- Continuing enjoyable activities
- Talking openly about your concerns
- Seeking help when needed

Emotional strength supports physical health.

The Role of Support

Support from others makes a real difference.

- Family can provide encouragement
- Friends offer emotional support
- Healthcare providers guide treatment

You do not have to manage arthritis alone.

Work and Daily Productivity

Many patients worry about their ability to work.

In most cases, with proper management:

- Work can continue
- Adjustments may be needed
- Short breaks improve efficiency
- Proper ergonomics reduce strain

Work provides not just income, but also purpose and confidence.

Adapting Without Losing Yourself

Arthritis may require changes in how you do things.

But change does not mean loss.

- You may move differently, but you can still move

- You may take more time, but you can still achieve your goals
- You may need help at times, but you remain capable

Adaptation is a sign of strength.

Doctor's Pearl

The patients who do best are not those who constantly fight their condition.

They are the ones who **understand it, accept it, and adapt wisely**.

Myth vs Fact

Myth: Arthritis means you must give up your normal life.
Fact: Most people continue active lives with proper care.

Myth: Flare-ups mean treatment has failed.
Fact: Flare-ups are common and manageable.

Common Mistakes to Avoid

- Overexerting on good days
- Stopping all activity on bad days
- Ignoring emotional health

- Avoiding social interaction
- Not asking for help

Red Flag Warnings

Seek medical advice if:

- Flare-ups become frequent or severe
- Daily activities become increasingly difficult
- Emotional distress becomes overwhelming
- Pain significantly disrupts sleep
- You feel unable to cope

Key Points

- Arthritis can be managed effectively
- Routine and consistency help
- Flare-ups are manageable
- Emotional health is important
- Independence can be preserved

Chapter Summary

Living well with arthritis requires a balanced approach
that includes physical activity, emotional well-being, and
practical adjustments. With understanding and
consistency, patients can remain active, independent, and
engaged in meaningful life activities.

Action Plan

- Create a simple daily routine
- Stay active with balanced movement
- Learn to manage flare-ups calmly
- Maintain social connections
- Seek support when needed
- Focus on long-term consistency

A Simple Real-Life Example

A patient once told me, "Doctor, I thought my life would become smaller because of arthritis."

Instead, with simple adjustments and consistent care, she continued to work, travel, and enjoy her family life.

She later said, "I did not lose my life. I just learned to live it differently."

Transition to the Next Chapter

Now that you understand how to live well with arthritis, the next step is to address common doubts.

In the next chapter, we will discuss **frequently asked questions and myths**, so you can move forward with clarity and confidence.

CHAPTER 18: Frequently Asked Questions and Myths – Clearing Confusion with Clarity

Why Clarity Matters So Much

Over the years, I have noticed something very consistent.

Patients do not struggle only with arthritis.
They also struggle with **confusion**.

Advice comes from many directions:

- Friends and relatives
- Internet searches
- Social media
- Half-understood medical discussions

Some of this information is useful. Much of it is misleading.

When information is unclear, decisions become uncertain. When decisions are uncertain, outcomes suffer.

This chapter is meant to do one simple but powerful thing.

Replace confusion with clarity.

Common Questions Patients Ask

Is arthritis curable?

For most types, the answer is no.

But that does not mean nothing can be done.

Arthritis can often be **controlled very effectively**. Many patients live active, comfortable lives.

Some inflammatory types may even go into remission with proper treatment.

Is arthritis only a disease of old age?

No.

While osteoarthritis is more common with age, many types of arthritis can occur in younger individuals.

Conditions like rheumatoid arthritis and ankylosing spondylitis often begin earlier in life.

Age is a risk factor, not the only cause.

Should I stop using a painful joint?

No.

Complete rest leads to stiffness and weakness.

The correct approach is **controlled movement**, not avoidance.

Does exercise worsen arthritis?

When done properly, no.

Exercise:

- Strengthens muscles
- Improves flexibility
- Reduces pain

The key is choosing the right type and doing it correctly.

Can diet cure arthritis?

Diet supports treatment, but it does not cure most forms.

It helps by:

- Reducing inflammation
- Controlling weight
- Improving overall health

It is an important part of management, not a complete solution.

Are pain medicines harmful?

When used correctly, they are safe and effective.

Problems arise when they are:

- Overused
- Used incorrectly
- Taken without proper guidance

Used wisely, they are helpful tools.

When should I see a specialist?

You should consider specialist care if:

- Diagnosis is uncertain
- Symptoms suggest inflammatory arthritis
- Pain is not controlled
- Advanced treatment is needed

Early consultation often leads to better outcomes.

Will I need surgery?

Not necessarily.

Many patients manage well without surgery.

Surgery is considered only when:

- Pain is severe
- Function is significantly limited
- Other treatments are not effective

Does weather affect arthritis?

Many patients report increased discomfort in cold or damp weather.

While the exact cause is not fully understood, this observation is common.

Can arthritis be prevented?

Not completely, but risk can be reduced.

Helpful measures include:

- Maintaining a healthy weight
- Staying active
- Avoiding joint injuries
- Managing other health conditions

Common Myths and the Reality

Myth: Arthritis means you must stop all activity

Reality: Movement is essential for joint health

Myth: Joint pain is always due to aging

Reality: Many forms occur in younger individuals

Myth: Cracking joints causes arthritis

Reality: There is no strong evidence to support this

Myth: Mild pain means mild disease

Reality: Some serious conditions begin with mild symptoms

Myth: Natural treatments are always safe

Reality: Some may have side effects or interact with medicines

---

Doctor's Pearl

Clear understanding reduces fear.

When you understand your condition, you take better control of it.

Common Mistakes to Avoid

- Believing unverified information
- Following advice without proper evaluation
- Ignoring medical guidance
- Delaying treatment
- Relying only on personal anecdotes

Red Flag Warnings

Seek medical advice if:

- You are unsure about your diagnosis
- Symptoms do not match expectations
- Treatment is not working
- You are considering alternative therapies
- You have unanswered concerns

Key Points

- Arthritis is manageable even if not curable
- Correct information is essential
- Many common beliefs are incorrect
- Treatment should be evidence-based
- Understanding improves confidence

Chapter Summary

Arthritis is often surrounded by myths and misconceptions. By understanding the facts and addressing common questions, patients can make informed decisions and manage their condition effectively. Clarity leads to confidence, and confidence leads to better outcomes.

Action Plan

- Ask questions during medical visits
- Verify information from reliable sources
- Avoid decisions based on myths
- Stay informed about your condition
- Follow evidence-based treatment plans

A Simple Real-Life Example

A patient stopped exercising because he believed it would worsen his arthritis.

Over time, his stiffness increased and his pain worsened.

After proper guidance, he resumed gentle exercise and improved significantly.

He later said, "Doctor, I wish I had known the truth earlier."

Transition to the Next Chapter

Now that we have addressed common doubts and misconceptions, it is time to bring everything together.

In the next chapter, we will focus on **long-term strategies to stay well**, so you can move forward with confidence and clarity.

CHAPTER 19: Staying Well Long-Term – Building a Life That Supports Your Joints

Thinking Beyond Today

By now, you understand arthritis much better.

You know what it is.
You know how it behaves.
You know how to manage it.

Now comes the most important question.

How do you stay well over the long term?

Arthritis is usually not a short-term problem. It is a condition that requires steady, thoughtful care over many years.

The encouraging part is this.

With the right approach, many patients remain active, independent, and satisfied with their quality of life.

Think Long-Term, Act Daily

One of the most common challenges I see is the expectation of quick results.

Patients try something for a short time and stop when they do not see immediate improvement.

But arthritis does not improve in a few days.

Progress comes from:

- Small steps
- Repeated consistently
- Over a long period

A short walk every day is more effective than a long walk once in a while.

Consistency is your greatest advantage.

Creating Your Personal Plan

There is no single plan that works for everyone.

Your approach should reflect:

- The type of arthritis you have
- Your age and overall health
- Your daily routine
- Your personal goals

However, most effective plans include:

- Regular physical activity
- Weight management
- Balanced nutrition
- Appropriate use of medicines

- Monitoring of symptoms

Think of this as your personal roadmap.

The Importance of Regular Follow-Up

Many patients feel better and stop follow-up visits.

This is a common mistake.

Regular follow-up helps to:

- Monitor disease progression
- Adjust treatment when needed
- Detect problems early
- Maintain motivation

Even when you feel well, staying connected with your doctor is important.

Preventing Flare-Ups

Flare-ups may still occur, but you can reduce their impact.

Helpful steps include:

- Recognizing early warning signs
- Adjusting activity levels early

- Using simple pain control methods
- Maintaining good sleep and stress habits

Prepared patients recover faster from flare-ups.

Staying Motivated Over Time

Long-term conditions can test your motivation.

There may be periods when progress feels slow.

During these times:

- Focus on small improvements
- Celebrate small successes
- Maintain your routine
- Remind yourself why you started

Motivation grows when you see steady progress.

The Role of Support

Support plays a major role in long-term success.

- Family encouragement helps maintain habits
- Friends provide emotional strength
- Healthcare providers guide treatment

You do not have to manage arthritis alone.

Adapting Without Losing Yourself

Arthritis may require changes in how you do things.

But change is not loss.

- You may move differently, but you can still move
- You may take more time, but you can still achieve your goals
- You may need help at times, but you remain capable

Adaptation is a strength, not a weakness.

Doctor's Pearl

The best outcomes come from partnership.

When patients and doctors work together with consistency and understanding, results are much better.

Myth vs Fact

Myth: Arthritis will inevitably lead to disability.
Fact: With proper care, many patients remain active and independent.

Myth: Medicines alone are enough.
Fact: Lifestyle and daily habits are equally important.

Common Mistakes to Avoid

- Expecting quick results
- Being inconsistent
- Skipping follow-up
- Ignoring early warning signs
- Losing motivation

Red Flag Warnings

Seek medical advice if:

- Symptoms worsen despite treatment
- New joints become involved
- Flare-ups become frequent
- Function declines
- Side effects occur

Key Points

- Arthritis requires long-term management
- Consistency is more important than intensity
- Personalized care improves outcomes
- Regular follow-up is essential
- Support systems help maintain success

Chapter Summary

Long-term success in managing arthritis depends on consistent daily habits, appropriate medical care, and regular follow-up. By focusing on small, sustainable changes and maintaining motivation, patients can preserve joint health and continue to lead active, fulfilling lives.

Action Plan

- Build a realistic daily routine
- Stay physically active
- Maintain a healthy weight
- Follow medical advice consistently
- Keep regular follow-up appointments
- Stay positive and focused

A Simple Real-Life Example

A patient once told me, "Doctor, I kept waiting for one treatment that would fix everything."

Over time, he realized that improvement came from many small steps.

Regular walking. Better eating. Consistent follow-up.

Years later, he remains active and independent.

Transition to the Final Chapter

You have now learned how to manage arthritis day by day and over the long term.

In the final chapter, we will bring everything together and focus on one simple and powerful message.

You are not defined by arthritis.

CHAPTER 20: Final Thoughts – Taking Charge of Your Health with Confidence

A Journey Toward Clarity

When you began this book, you may have had many questions.

What is happening to my joints?
Will this get worse?
What can I do about it?

These are natural concerns.

Now, as you reach the end, I hope something has changed.

You now have **clarity**.

You understand what arthritis is, how it develops, how it is diagnosed, and how it can be managed.

That understanding is powerful.

From Uncertainty to Confidence

One of the greatest burdens of arthritis is not just pain.

It is uncertainty.

When we do not understand a condition, we tend to worry more, delay action, and lose confidence.

But knowledge changes that.

When you understand your condition:

- You recognize symptoms early
- You take appropriate steps
- You avoid unnecessary fear
- You make informed decisions

Confidence grows when confusion fades.

You Have More Control Than You Think

It is easy to feel that arthritis is something that simply happens to you.

But that is not the whole story.

You may not control every aspect of the disease.

But you do control many important factors:

- Your activity level
- Your weight
- Your daily habits
- Your consistency
- Your approach to treatment

These choices have a real impact on your outcome.

I have seen patients with similar conditions have very different results, simply because of how they managed their health.

Small Steps, Meaningful Change

You do not need to change everything at once.

In fact, trying to do too much too quickly often leads to frustration.

A better approach is simple:

- Start small
- Stay consistent
- Build gradually

A short walk each day.
A small improvement in diet.
A simple stretching routine.

Over time, these small steps create meaningful change.

The Importance of Partnership

Managing arthritis is not something you do alone.

A strong partnership with your doctor is essential.

- Share your symptoms clearly
- Ask questions
- Follow treatment plans
- Report concerns early

When patients and doctors work together, outcomes improve.

Living a Full and Meaningful Life

It is important to remember this clearly.

You are more than your arthritis.

Your life includes:

- Your family
- Your work
- Your interests
- Your goals

Arthritis may require adjustments, but it does not take away your ability to live a full and meaningful life.

Doctor's Pearl

Perfection is not required.

Consistency is.

Myth vs Fact

Myth: Arthritis always leads to disability.
Fact: With proper care, many patients remain active and independent.

Myth: Nothing can be done.
Fact: There are many effective ways to manage arthritis.

Common Mistakes to Avoid

- Waiting too long to act
- Expecting quick fixes
- Being inconsistent
- Ignoring follow-up
- Losing hope

Red Flag Reminder

Even as you move forward, seek medical advice if:

- Symptoms worsen suddenly
- New joints become involved
- Function declines
- New or unusual symptoms appear

Early action always helps.

Key Points

- Understanding reduces fear
- You have meaningful control over your health
- Small, consistent steps lead to success
- Partnership with your doctor improves outcomes
- Arthritis does not define your life

Chapter Summary

Arthritis is a manageable condition when approached with knowledge, consistency, and a balanced mindset. By understanding the disease and taking steady, practical steps, patients can maintain mobility, independence, and quality of life. Confidence replaces fear when clarity is achieved.

Action Plan

- Start with one small change today
- Stay consistent with daily habits
- Follow medical advice regularly
- Maintain a positive and realistic outlook
- Focus on long-term health

A Final Reflection

Over many years of practice, I have seen patients take very different paths.

Some waited, hoping for a quick cure.

Others took small, steady steps and stayed consistent.

The second group almost always did better.

The difference was not the disease.

The difference was the approach.

A Closing Message

If there is one message I want you to carry forward, it is this:

You can live well with arthritis.

Not by ignoring it.
Not by fearing it.
But by understanding it, respecting it, and managing it wisely.

Take one step today.

Then another tomorrow.

Over time, those steps will lead you to a healthier, more active, and more confident life.

APPENDIX A: A Simple Daily Routine for Arthritis Care

Why a Daily Routine Makes a Difference

In my experience, patients who follow a simple, steady routine do far better than those who rely only on occasional effort.

Arthritis responds to **consistency, not intensity**.

You do not need a complicated plan. You need a realistic routine that fits your life and that you can follow every day.

A Practical Day Plan

Morning

- Wake up at a regular time
- Begin with gentle stretching for 5 to 10 minutes
- Take a warm shower if stiffness is significant
- Eat a balanced breakfast
- Take prescribed medicines as advised

Morning is the time when stiffness is usually highest. Gentle movement helps loosen joints and prepares you for the day.

Midday

- Stay active with normal daily tasks
- Avoid long periods of sitting or standing
- Take short breaks every 30 to 45 minutes
- Maintain good posture during work
- Drink adequate water

Balance is important. Avoid both overexertion and prolonged inactivity.

Evening

- Engage in light physical activity such as walking
- Perform simple strengthening exercises
- Avoid heavy or strenuous activity late in the day
- Eat a balanced dinner

Evening activity helps maintain mobility without overloading joints.

Night

- Wind down with relaxation techniques
- Maintain a regular sleep schedule
- Use comfortable pillows and joint support
- Avoid stimulants late in the evening

Good sleep supports recovery and reduces pain
sensitivity.

Key Points

- Keep the routine simple
- Stay consistent
- Adjust based on your condition
- Avoid extremes

APPENDIX B: Simple Home Exercises You Can Start Safely

Why Exercise at Home Matters

Regular exercise does not require a gym.

Simple movements performed correctly at home can:

- Improve flexibility
- Strengthen muscles
- Reduce stiffness
- Support joint health

Basic Exercises

Gentle Stretching

- Neck movements: slow side-to-side and forward-back
- Shoulder rolls
- Finger opening and closing
- Ankle rotations

Perform slowly and avoid sudden movements.

Strengthening Exercises

- Sit-to-stand from a chair
- Straight leg raises
- Light resistance band exercises
- Wall push-ups

Start with a few repetitions and increase gradually.

Low-Impact Activity

- Walking
- Stationary cycling
- Water-based exercises if available

Aim for regular activity rather than occasional intense sessions.

Safety Tips

- Start slowly
- Stop if you feel sharp pain
- Maintain proper form
- Stay consistent

APPENDIX C: Foods That Support Joint Health

A Practical Approach to Eating

You do not need a complicated diet plan.

Focus on **simple, balanced eating habits**.

Helpful Foods

- Fresh fruits and vegetables
- Whole grains
- Nuts and seeds
- Fish rich in omega-3
- Legumes such as beans and lentils
- Healthy oils like olive oil

Foods to Limit

- Processed foods
- Excess sugar
- Sugary drinks
- Excess red and processed meat
- Refined carbohydrates

Hydration

- Drink adequate water throughout the day
- Stay especially well hydrated in gout

Key Principle

Consistency matters more than perfection.

APPENDIX D: When to Seek Medical Help

Do Not Delay When It Matters

Many patients wait too long before seeking help.

Recognizing warning signs early can prevent complications.

Seek Medical Advice If You Notice

- Persistent joint pain lasting weeks
- Swelling, warmth, or redness
- Morning stiffness lasting more than one hour
- Sudden severe joint pain
- Difficulty walking or performing daily tasks
- Joint pain with fever

Regular Follow-Up Is Important

Even if symptoms improve:

- Continue follow-up visits

- Review treatment plans
- Monitor for side effects
- Adjust therapy when needed

APPENDIX E: Your Personal Arthritis Tracker

Why Tracking Helps

Patients who track their symptoms understand their condition better.

This helps in:

- Identifying patterns
- Recognizing flare-ups early
- Improving communication with your doctor

What to Track Daily

- Pain level (scale of 1 to 10)
- Morning stiffness duration
- Swelling or redness
- Activity level
- Sleep quality
- Medications taken

What to Review Weekly

- Overall improvement or worsening

- Frequency of flare-ups
- Ability to perform daily activities

Keep It Simple

Use a notebook or a simple digital note.

Do not make it complicated.

The goal is awareness, not perfection.

Thank You and Please Review the Book

Thank you for taking the time to read this book. I sincerely hope it has helped you understand your health a little more clearly and has given you practical, everyday steps you can follow with confidence. If you found this book helpful, **I would truly appreciate it if you could leave a brief and honest review.** Even a few lines sharing your experience can make a meaningful difference. Your feedback helps other readers find reliable, trustworthy health information and supports them in making better decisions for themselves and their families.

Warm regards,

Dr Prabhat Das

Continue your Healthcare Journey with these Books

Good health is a journey, not a single step. It is not achieved in one day or with one book. That is why I created the "Better Health with Dr Das Series", with each book addressing a different common condition. If you would like easy, practical guidance on other everyday health concerns, you may wish to explore the rest of books in this series.

Books in this series:

- Better Health starts Here: A Doctor's Guide to Staying Healthy After 40
- A Doctor's Easy Guide to Understanding & Managing OBESITY
- Doctor, What DIET Is Best for Me?
- Doctor, Why Can't I Lose Weight? A Doctor's Guide to Safe & Sustainable Weight Loss)
- A Doctor's Easy Guide to GLP-1 for Obesity
- A Doctor's Easy Guide to Understanding & Managing HIGH BLOOD PRESSURE
- A Doctor's Guide to Living Well With DIABETES
- A Doctor's Guide to Understanding & Managing THYROID DISEASES
- A Doctor's Guide to Understanding & Managing HIGH CHOLESTEROL
- A Doctor's Practical Guide to HEART HEALTH After 40: How to Protect Your Heart & Live Longer
- A Doctor's Guide to Healing & Reversing FATTY LIVER DISEASE: Simple, Natural & Science-Based Steps to Reduce Liver Fat and Prevent Complications

- Control <u>Your ACID REFLUX, HEARTBURN &</u> <u>GERD</u>: A Doctor's Practical Guide that Works
- Live Comfortably with <u>IRRITABLE BOWEL</u> <u>SYNDROME:</u> A Doctor's Practical Guide to Understanding & Managing <u>IBS</u>
- A Doctor's Practical Guide to Understanding & Managing <u>GALLBLADDER STONES & OTHER</u> <u>PROBLEMS</u>
- Take Control of <u>COPD:</u> A Doctor's Practical Guide to Better Breathing
- Living Better with <u>ASTHMA:</u> A Doctor's Practical Guide to Asthma Control
- <u>SLEEP APNEA, INSOMNIA & OTHER SLEEP</u> <u>DISORDERS:</u> A Doctor's Practical Guide to Better Sleep & Better Health
- Protect Your <u>KIDNEYS:</u> A Doctor's Practical Guide to Kidney Health & Prevention
- <u>PROSTATE HEALTH</u>: A Doctor's Practical Guide to Early Detection & Care
- <u>ARTHRITIS:</u> A Doctor's Practical Guide to Pain Control & Mobility
- A Doctor's Practical Guide to Fixing <u>BACK PAIN</u> Step by Step
- <u>COMMON SKIN & HAIR PROBLEMS:</u> A Doctor's Practical Guide to Skin & Hair Care
- <u>DEMENTIA & MEMORY LOSS</u>: A Doctor's Practical Guide to Prevention & Management
- Doctor, Why Am I <u>TIRED</u> All the Time? Fixing Fatigue & Getting Your Energy Back